The effect of the Reaset Approach

ISBN: 1537212915
ISBN-13: 978-1537212913

Thesis for obtaining the title:
Bachelor of Science in Osteopathy

The effect of the Reaset Approach

on the autonomic nervous system, state-trait anxiety and musculoskeletal pain in patients with work-related stress: A pilot study

TOM MEYERS

ABSTRACT

Background: Work-related stress (WRS) is associated with musculoskeletal pain (MSP), changes in the autonomic nervous system (ANS) and anxiety.

Objective: To determine the feasibility of a follow-up study and treatment efficacy of the Reaset Approach on MSP, ANS and State-Trait anxiety.

Methods: 15 subjects with WRS and MSP were assigned into 3 groups (Body, Head-Neck, Head-Neck-Body). Each group received a single 25 minute 'Reaset Approach' intervention. Heart rate variability (HRV), electro-dermal activity (EDA), State Trait Anxiety (STAI) and MSP were measured.

Results: HRV parameters: SDNN increased in 13 of 15 subjects while SD1 and SD2 increased in 12 of 15 subjects. EDA reduced in 10 of 14 subjects. State Anxiety reduced in all subjects and Trait Anxiety reduced in 14 of 15 subjects. MSP reduced in all subjects after the intervention and were still lower three days afterwards.

Conclusions: This pilot study determined that a follow-up study can ensue provided minor modifications are implemented and that the 'Reaset Approach' has an influence on the ANS, anxiety and MSP. Results do differ between groups. The intervention groups including the head and neck modalities demonstrated better results.

Keywords: Osteopathy, work-related stress, state-trait anxiety, autonomic nervous system, musculoskeletal pain, SF-MPQ, STAI, EDA, HRV

I. TABLE OF CONTENTS

II.   FIGURES

III. TABLES

DISCLAIMER

The information provided in this book is designed to provide helpful information on the subjects discussed. This book is not meant to be used, nor should it be used, to diagnose or treat any medical condition. For diagnosis or treatment of any medical problem, consult your own physician. The publisher and author are not responsible for any specific health or allergy needs that may require medical supervision and are not liable for any damages or negative consequences from any treatment, action, application or preparation, to any person reading or following the information in this book. References are provided for informational purposes only and do not constitute endorsement of any websites or other sources. Readers should be aware that the websites listed in this book may change.

DECLARATION OF CONFORMITY

I declare that this dissertation is the product of my own work, that it has not been submitted before for any degree or examination in any other university, and that all the sources I have used or quoted have been indicated and acknowledged as complete references.

Signature:

Tom Meyers

Osteopathie Schule Deutschland

Dresden International University

Examiners: Dipl.-Ing. Bettina Thiel and Dr., MSc Ost. Tobias Schmid

1 INTRODUCTION

Work-related (psychosocial) stress considered to be one of the greatest health challenges in Europe, is on the rise. It is estimated that 1 in 4 workers is affected by work-related stress, and that it contributes to 50-60% of sick days, with an annual economic cost of up to €20 billion in the EU15 (EU-OSHA, 2009).

Work-related stress is experienced when the demands of the work environment exceed the employee's ability to cope with them (EU-OSHA, 2007). Work-related stress is associated with musculoskeletal disorders (Eurofound, 2007), changes in the autonomic nervous system (ANS) (Chandola, 2010) as evidenced by an increase in electro-dermal activity (EDA) (Setz, 2010) and the decrease of heart-rate variability (HRV) (Hjortskov *et al.*, 2004), (Brosschot, *et al.*, 2007), (Kang *et al.*, 2004).

Lowered HRV is associated with anxiety (Friendman, 2007) (Licht *et al.*, 2009) (Alvares *et al*, 2013), cardiovascular disease (Task Force of The European Society of Cardiology and The North American Society of Pacing and Electrophysiology, 1996) and chronic musculoskeletal pain (Macfarlane *et al.*, 2009). There is also a relationship between low HRV and increased cortisol levels, which in turn is associated with decreased cognitive performance (Johnson *et al.*, 2012)

Increase in HRV regulation is associated with emotional regulation (Thayer and Lane, 2009) and cognitive performance, and thus improved work performance (Hansen, *et al.*, 2003).

A small number of studies have shown that osteopathic manipulative treatment (OMT) has an influence on the autonomic nervous system and increase in HRV when performed, for example, in the cervical region (Henley, 2008) and sub-occipital region (Giles, 2013).

It has come to the attention of the investigator that patients with non-trauma related musculoskeletal pain (MSP) and self-declared work stress have reported pain relief, reduced anxiety levels, improved cognitive performance and stress reduction after one 'Reaset Approach' treatment, an osteopathic functional method approach.

The investigator is interested to know whether a relationship can be determined between the Reaset Approach and reduced musculoskeletal pain, stress and anxiety levels.

2 BACKGROUND

The evolution towards a more computerized work environment has changed the way we work and the way work is organized today. These changes have given rise to new occupational health and safety risks, adding psychosocial risks on top of the existing physical and biological risks (EU-OSHA, 2007). A survey by the European Foundation for the Improvement of Living and Working Conditions identified that musculoskeletal pain and stress at work as the most common threats from the working environment (EUROFOUND, 2007).

2.1 WORK-RELATED MUSCULOSKELETAL PAIN

Musculoskeletal pain is the foremost health threat posed by the working environment. In a computerized work environment this is generally ascribed to poor workstation ergonomics, high workload, limited variation in work, and typing style (Punnet, Bergqvist, 1997). However, a systematic review by Waersted, Hanvold and Veiersted (2010) focusing on the specific physical factors involved in computer work concluded that there is limited epidemiological evidence for associating these physical factors of computer work with musculoskeletal disorders. Similarly, Andersen et al. (2010) concluded that there is no clear causal association between upper extremity disorders and computer use. However, they did point out that the reviews indicated an association between pain complaints and intense computer use.

Psychological and psychosocial factors have been shown more conclusively to contribute to work-related musculoskeletal symptoms (Jensen, et al., 2002) (Griffiths, Mackey, Adamson, 2007). In an evaluation of review articles for consistency in conclusions, the European League Against Rheumatism (EULAR) Task Force (Macfarlane, et al., 2009) also confirmed the association between work-related psychosocial factors and musculoskeletal pain. However, the EULAR Task Force does point out that many reviews reached different conclusions depending on what was evaluated, and how the evidence was assessed (Macfarlane, et al., 2009).

Griffiths, Mackey and Adamson (2007) posit an interactive relationship between biomechanics, psychological and psychosocial demands, and that their combination has a greater influence on musculoskeletal symptoms than the sum of its parts. This threefold interaction is known as the biopsychosocial model and widely accepted as the most heuristic approach to chronic pain (Gatchel, et al., 2007).

2.2 WORK-RELATED STRESS

Work-related stress is the second most common health problem at work (EUROFOUND, 2007). In 2005 stress was experienced by 22% of EU workers (EU-OSHA, 2009).

Work-related stress is experienced when the demands of the work environment exceeds the employee's ability to cope with them (EU-OSHA, 2007). It is directly linked to the increase of emerging psychosocial risks due to poor work design, organization and management, as well as a poor social context of work (EU-OSHA, 2009). These are, in turn, the result of the implementation of new processes, new technologies, new types of workplaces and social or organizational changes.

Stress, and psychosocial stress in particular, has been linked with changes in the autonomic nervous system (Jarczok, 2013) (Petrowski, et al. 2010) and the HPA axis. Chronic psychosocial stress has a detrimental effect on health (Korte, et al. 2005). Such effects range from muscle tissue atrophy, impairment of growth and tissue repair and suppression of the immune system, to alterations of brain structures - all conditions that contribute to the development and maintenance of a variety of chronic pain conditions (Gatchel, 2007) and musculoskeletal pain (Jensen, et al., 2002) (Griffiths, Mackey, Adamson, 2007).

Stress-induced changes in the autonomic nervous system, with reduced parasympathetic activity and/or increase sympathetic activity as demonstrated by HRV, are indicated as the reason why work-related stress leads to musculoskeletal pain and the maintenance of the musculoskeletal pain itself (Jarczok, et al., 2013) (Hallman, Ekman and Lyskov, 2013). Changes in autonomic nervous system balance is furthermore associated with anxiety disorders. (Chalmers, et al., 2014).

2.3 OSTEOPATHY AND THE AUTONOMIC NERVOUS SYSTEM

Osteopathic Manipulative Treatment (OMT) is best known for its efficacy on musculoskeletal disorders especially low-back pain (Licciardone, Brimhall and King, 2005) (Licciardone, et al., 2013). OMT is also used for non-musculoskeletal conditions like trauma, neurologic, respiratory, cardiovascular and gastrointestinal (Johnson and Kurtz, 2002) and conditions that are related to autonomic nervous system disorders. Henley, et al. (2008) demonstrated the relationship between OMT involving a cervical myofascial release and the autonomic nervous system in a repeated measures study with healthy subjects.

A pilot study by Girsberger, et al, (2014) on the influence of a 30-minute craniosacral treatment on the autonomic nervous system showed a more significant increase in SDNN and Total Power (TP) compared the control rest period.

2.4 STRESS, PAIN AND OSTEOPATHY

Stress is a natural survival response of the body. However, chronic biological, psychological (psychosocial) stress is detrimental to health and seen as an important cause of musculoskeletal pain in low back and shoulder/neck pain (Mcfarlane, et al., 2009).

Chronic stress also changes the neurophysiological balance, which in turn has an influence on blood vessels, healing efficacy, posture (Finestone, Alfceli and Fisher, 2008), brain structure and behavior, leading to pain, illness and disease.

The question that arises is how often the chronic musculoskeletal pain bringing patients to an osteopath (Johnson and Kurtz, 2002) is related to stress (Mcfarlane, 2007). Musculoskeletal pain that has as an onset a cascade of biopsychosocially induced changes in neurophysiology (Finestone, Alfeeli and Fisher, 2008) benefits from a biopsychosocial treatment model. Is osteopathy such an approach?

According to Penny (2010), the biopsychosocial model of pain is in line with the 4 currently accepted osteopathic tenets: Body is a unit capable of self-regulation; self-healing and health maintenance, structure and function are reciprocally interrelated; and that a rational treatment is based on the above the basic principles of body unity, self-regulation, and the interrelationship of structure and function.

In this study, the investigator will test the effect of the 'Reaset Approach' - a novel functional method based on the osteopathic principles - on the autonomic nervous system, state and trait anxiety levels and musculoskeletal pain in subjects with work-related stress.

The term 'Reaset' is a fusion of the words 'reset' and 'ease'. Reset is used in the sense of bringing a system to its normal condition (Merriam-Webster). Ease refers to freedom from pain or trouble, comfort of body or mind (Merriam-Webster) and being comfortable and free from stress (Wiktionary).

'Approach' is used as meaning 'a way of dealing with' (Oxford) and chosen instead of 'technique' to address the underlying notion that it is based on a dynamic principle and not a fixed modality.

RA is considered a functional method (AACOM, 2011), an indirect treatment approach consisting of three phases: the engagement (E) phase involves placing the hands on a portion of the patient's body and - in response to the sensation of the movement that is perceived - passively accompanying the tissues towards their dynamic balance point. Stage two is holding the position of balanced tension (O) and allowing for spontaneous readjustment or release, which is the third stage (D).

The practitioner's attention is focused on the palpatory feedback, stays neutral, non-judgmental and does not search for a cause or dysfunction. The practitioner is there to catalyze the self-regulatory and self-healing mechanisms, thereby bringing ease in tissue and articulations.

The subjects remain supine and passive during all three phases of the RA approach.

3 QUESTIONS

This pilot study was conducted in order to evaluate feasibility and identify any modifications needed in the design of an ensuing randomized controlled trial to test and compare the effect of the novel 'Reaset Approach' in 3 different interventions on the autonomic nervous system, self-reported state and trait an anxiety levels and self-assessed perceived musculoskeletal pain.

The secondary objective was to get preliminary treatment effect results in the 3 groups:

- Body (B)
- Head and neck (HN)
- Head, Neck and Body (HNB)

3.1 FEASIBILITY

- Is it possible to recruit enough subjects for a larger study with the current eligibility criteria?
- Are the questionnaires understandable to the subjects?
- Are there any unforeseen difficulties in the management of this study?
- Can the study site handle the number of subjects foreseen for the larger study?
- Are there any major issues with the handling of the data?

3.2 TREATMENT EFFECT

- Does the Reaset Approach influence ANS activity and is there a difference between the 3 intervention groups?

- Does the 'Reaset Approach' influence state and trait anxiety and is there a difference between the 3 intervention groups?

- Does the 'Reaset Approach' influence perceived musculoskeletal pain and is there a difference between the 3 intervention groups?

4 METHODS

4.1 STUDY DESIGN

This pilot study was a single-intervention, randomized clinical trial to provide main trial feasibility and preliminary evidence of treatment efficacy.

Subjects were randomly assigned to a group and received a single intervention of 25 minutes using the Reset Approach. The three groups were:

B: 'Reset Approach' on body

HN: 'Reset Approach' on head and neck

HNB: 'Reset Approach' on head, neck and body

Three treatment effects were assessed in view of the main study: autonomic nervous system, anxiety levels and musculoskeletal pain.

The autonomic nervous system was indirectly evaluated for 5 minutes before (t1) and after (t2) the intervention with the Biosign® "HRV-Scanner" and the MentalBioScreen 'K3' for EDA values.

Anxiety was measured using the State-Trait Anxiety Inventory (STAI). Trait anxiety was self-assessed 1 to 3 days before (t0) and 3 weeks after (t4) the intervention. State anxiety was assessed just before and immediately after the intervention.

Musculoskeletal pain was assessed with the Short-Form McGill Pain Questionnaire (SF-MPQ) just before (t1), right after (t2) and 3 days after (t3) the intervention.

Table 1: Organizational Chart

STAY Y-2: Trait Anxiety, STAI Y-1: State Anxiety, SF-MPQ: Short-Form McGill Pain Questionnaire, HRV: Heart Rate Variability, EDA: Electro Dermal Activity, B: Body, HN: Head and Neck, HNB: Head, Neck and Body

≤ 3 day(s)	Trial day of visit										+ 3 days	+21 days
t0	t1	t1			t1	Intervention	t2		t2	t2	t3	t4
STAI Y-2	STAI Y-1	SF MPQ	Set up	Rest	HRV EDA	B/HN/HNB	HRV EDA	End	STAI Y-1	SF MPQ	SF MPQ	STAI Y-2
(I)	(I)	(I)							(II)	(II)	(III)	(I)
6 min.	6 min.	4 min.	7 min.	5 min.	5 min.	25 min.	5 min.	3 min.	6 min.	4 min.	4 min.	6 min.

4.2 PARTICIPANTS

42 subjects were recruited through referral, newsletters, emails, announcements on radio and social networks.

Subjects were screened by means of a structured telephone interview (Add. 9.3) to ensure that their characteristics match a list of admission criteria.

4.2.1 INCLUSION CRITERIA

- Subjects aged between 30 and 50 years
- Perceived work-related stress higher than 6 on a 11-point numeric rating scale
- Experiencing musculoskeletal tension or pain

All subjects had to meet all three inclusion criteria.

4.2.2 EXCLUSION CRITERIA

- Use of medication: antidepressants, psychotropic medication, sleeping pills, muscle relaxants or medication for heart or blood pressure.
- Psychiatric illness or psychosis
- Heart problems
- Allergies
- Diabetes
- Operation in the last 12 months
- Pregnancy or suspected pregnancy
- Menopause
- Previously treated by the investigator

Subjects were asked to abstain from smoking, drinking caffeinated drinks, consuming food or alcohol 2 hours prior to the intervention. All subjects complied.

4.2.3 RECRUITMENT

After the structured telephone interview, 27 subjects were excluded for not meeting all of the inclusion or exclusion criteria, leaving 15 subjects to take part in the pilot study. The main reasons for exclusion were insufficient knowledge of the English language, no current musculoskeletal pain, or -related stress below 6 on the numeric rating scale during the structured telephone interview.

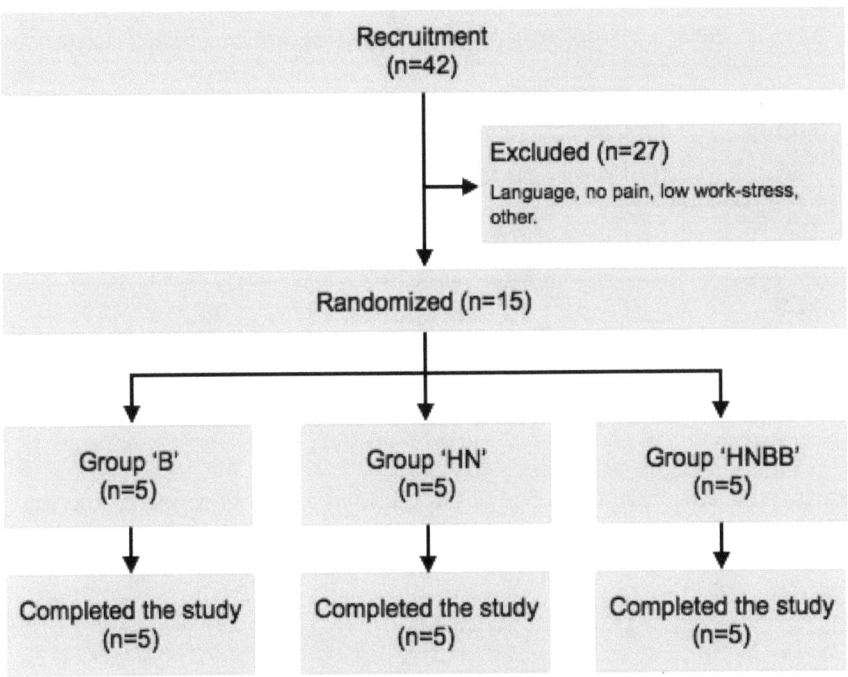

Figure 1: Flow diagram from recruitment to end of study

In total 13 women (87%) and 2 men (13%) aged between 33 and 47 were included in the study.

The subjects self-assessed perceived work-related stress level lay between 6 and 9 and was measured using a NRS, '0' indicating no perceived work-related stress to '10' the worst imaginable perceived work-related stress.

Table 2: Demographical data summary

Gender, age, work-related stress level (Numeric Rating Scale: 0-10) for each group

Group	Gender (F=Female - M=Male)	Age (min-max)	Work-Stress (min-max)
B	5 F	33-47	7-9
HN	5 F	33-44	6-9
HNB	3 F + 2 M	37-40	6-8

During the structured interview, all included subjects reported having muscular tension or pain.

Table 3: Subject group allocation and demographical data

Subject identification (ID),
Group allocation: B = Body; HN: Head and Neck; Head, Neck and Body
Subject gender: 1 = female; 0 = male
Handedness: R= right handed; L= left handed
Age in years
Weight in kg, height in m, BMI
Work-related stress level: Numeric Rating Scale: 0-10, prior to the appointment (t0).

ID	Group	Gender	Age	Handed	Weight	Height	BMI	Stress t0
1	B	1	47	R	61	1,64	22,7	8
2	HNB	1	40	R	62	1,79	19,4	6
3	HN	1	36	R	67	1,68	23,7	7
4	HNB	0	36	R	82	1,96	21,3	7
5	B	1	33	R	60	1,63	22,6	7
6	B	1	34	L	57	1,7	19,7	7
7	HNB	1	38	R	60	1,6	23,4	8
8	HN	1	33	R	63	1,69	22,1	6
9	HNB	1	38	R	55	1,63	20,7	6
10	HNB	0	37	R	75	1,77	23,9	/
11	B	1	34	R	50	1,65	18,4	7
12	HN	1	44	R	52	1,65	19,1	9
13	B	1	38	R	60	1,5	26,7	9
14	HN	1	40	R	55	1,63	20,7	8
15	HN	1	36	R	65	1,6	25,4	6
Mean			37,6		61,6	1,7	22,0	7,2
SD			3,94		8,37	0,11	2,40	1,01

4.2.4 RANDOMIZATION

In advance of the study, the investigator prepared a black cotton bag containing 15 folded pieces of paper, 5 showing 'B' for the intervention on the body, 5 showing 'HN' for the intervention on head and neck and 5 showing 'HNB' for the head, neck and body intervention group.

2 minutes before the start of each intervention, the investigator picked 1 folded coded piece of paper out of the black cotton bag. The intervention mentioned was the one the investigator applied.

4.3 PARAMETERS

In this pilot study the possible influence on the autonomic nervous system was indirectly evaluated through HRV and EDA measurements. State and Trait anxiety was measured with the STAI-forms and musculoskeletal pain was measured with the SF-MPQ.

4.3.1 HEART RATE VARIABILITY

The HRV measurements in this study were registered with the Biosign® "HRV-Scanner on the basis of a 5-minute electrocardiography (ECG) reading recorded immediately before (t1) and after (t2) the intervention with 2 electrodes on the chest.

For this study the following HRV parameters were used:

SDNN (ms): The standard deviation of the NN intervals reflects all the cyclic components responsible for variability in the period of recording.

SD1 (ms): Describes the scattering of the heart beats in the Poincaré diagram, reflects the width of the scatter plot and contains more information about fast-reacting changes of the heart rate or short-term variability (Piskorski and Guzik, 2005).

SD2 (ms): Describes the scattering of the heartbeats in the Poincaré diagram, expresses the length of the scatter plot and reflects both short-term and long-term variability (Piskorski and Guzik, 2005).

4.3.2 ELECTRO-DERMAL ACTIVITY

EDA was measured with the MentalBioScreen 'K3' for 5 minutes before (t1) and after (t2) the intervention with 2 electrodes placed on the hypothenar of the non-dominant hand.

4.3.3 STATE ANXIETY

State anxiety was measured with the State-Trait Anxiety Inventory Y-1 form (STAI Y-1) consisting of 20 statements to evaluate how subjects feel immediately before (t1) and after (t2) the intervention. Subjects were instructed to evaluate the different statements by circling one of the appropriate numbers to the right of the statement: 1 = not at all, 2 = somewhat, 3 = moderately so, 4 = very much so. (Add. 9.8)

The investigator scored the form using the appropriate Y-1 scoring-key supplied with the license (Add. 9.7). The weighted scores were then added to form a total STAI Y-1 score, which could vary from a minimum of 20 to a maximum of 80.

4.3.4 TRAIT ANXIETY

State anxiety was measured with the State Trait Anxiety Inventory Y-2 form (STAI Y-2) and consists of 20 statements to evaluate how subjects feet in general (over the last 3 weeks) 1 to 3 days before (t0) and 3 weeks after (t4) the intervention. Subjects were instructed to evaluate the different statements by circling one of the appropriate numbers to the right of the statement: 1 = almost never, 2 = sometimes, 3 = often, 4 = almost always.

The investigator scored the form by using the appropriate Y-2 form scoring-key supplied with the license. The weighted scores were then added up to form a total STAI Y-2 score, which could vary from a minimum of 20 to a maximum of 80.

4.3.5 PERCEIVED PAIN

Perceived pain was measure just before (t1), immediately after (t2) and 3 days (t3) after the intervention, using the SF-MPQ.

The SF-MPQ used for this study included:

- An outline of a human body, front and back: Subjects were asked to mark the location of current pain points
- A VAS: Subjects were asked to make a mark on the line that represented their current pain intensity
- A Present Pain Intensity (PPI) scale (E): Subjects were asked to read the 5 verbal descriptors (0 = no pain, 1 = mild, 2 = discomforting, 3 = distressing, 4 = horrible and 5 = excruciating) and indicate one that they felt described their current pain intensity best.
- Quality-of-pain score: A list of 15 words describing various qualities of pain, of which 11 represented the sensory (S) and 4 the affective (A) dimension of the pain experience. Subjects were asked to score each dimension none (blank, no indication), mild, moderate or severe.

The VAS pain intensity was determined by measuring in millimeters the distance from the no pain mark to the subject's mark. When the actual length of the VAS was distorted after scanning and printing (Snow and Kirwan, 1988) the measured distance was divided by the actual length of the line and multiplied by 10.

The total SF-MPQ score (T) was measured by adding up the S, A and E scores (T= S+A+E).

4.4 MEASURING INSTRUMENTS

4.4.1 HEART RATE VARIABILITY

Short-term 5-minute HRV was measured with the Biosign® "HRV-Scanner".

The HRV scanner is a protection class III device, compliant with EN 60335-1 and the relevant EC ordinances confirmed by the EC declaration of conformity (BioSign, 2012).

The electrodes used were W 55GS, press stud, 55 mm diameter, structurevlies with an acrylic adhesive, Ag/Ag/Cl sensor, hydro special solid gel ordered from the company Hasomed®. The electrodes had an offset voltage of 1,2 mV and impedance of 345 Ohm.

Measurements were in compliance with the Task Force of the European Society of Cardiology and North American Society of Pacing and Electrophysiology (1996).

4.4.2 ELECTRO-DERMAL ACTIVITY

EDA was measured using the MentalBioScreen 'K3', a CE class IIa certified medical devise from the company Porta Bio Screen© GmbH. The MentalBioScreen 'K3', is an exosomatic measuring tool with alternating current.

The electrodes used were the W 55GS, press stud, 55 mm diameter, structurevlies with an acrylic adhesive, Ag/Ag/Cl sensor, hydro special solid gel ordered from the company Hasomed®. The electrodes had an offset voltage of 1,2 mV and impedance of 345 Ohm.

4.4.3 STATE-TRAIT ANXIETY INVENTORY

The STAI form Y-1 and Y-2 are self-evaluation questionnaires for measuring, respectively, state and trait anxiety. The questionnaires, developed by Charles Spielberger (1983), have been used in over 8000 studies (Groth-Marnat, 2003). Average reliability coefficients are acceptable for internal consistency and test–retest reliability (Barnes, Harp and Jung, 2002), (Spielberger, 1983).

The STAI for adults reproduction license was obtained on 25 March 2014.

4.4.4 SHORT-FORM MCGILL PAIN QUESTIONNAIRE

The Short-Form McGill Pain Questionnaire (SF-MPQ) is a self-administered questionnaire developed by R. Melzack which measures subjective evaluation of sensory, affective and overall intensity of pain (Melzack, 1987). The questionnaire has been shown to be reliable, valid and consistent (Strand, et al., 2008).

Dr. Melzack authorized the use of the questionnaire by email on 21 January 2014.

4.5 INTERVENTIONS

The interventions were based on a novel treatment method called 'Reaset Approach' (RA) and was developed by the investigator.

4.5.1 INTERVENTION 'B': BODY

The RA was applied on the body for 25 minutes. The investigator placed his hands or fingers and applied the EOD phases as describe above (2.4) until release was perceived on the following parts of the body and in the following order: arm - shoulder (left and right), forearm (left and right), diaphragm, liver cylinder, kidney cylinder (left and right), caecum cylinder, stomach cylinder, sigmoid cylinder, hip joint (left and right), knee (left and right), ankle (left and right), fibula (left and right), feet (left and right), sacrum and sacrum–spine (Figure 2). The investigator went through the routine a second time and applied the RA again when needed. (Cylinders are as described by Fiew, L. and Ott, M., 2005)

4.5.2 INTERVENTION 'HN': HEAD AND NECK

The RA was applied on head and neck for 25 minutes. The practitioner placed his hands or fingers and applied the EOD phases as described above until release was perceived on the following parts of the cranium and in the following order: occipital bone, mastoid bone, sphenoid bone, parietal bone, frontal bone - occipital bone and along the neck (Figure 3). The investigator went through the routine a second time and applied the RA again when needed.

4.5.3 INTERVENTION 'HNB': HEAD, NECK AND BODY

The RA was applied on head, neck (Figure 2) and subsequently the body (Figure 3) as described above for 25 minutes. The investigator went through the routine a second time and applied the RA again when needed.

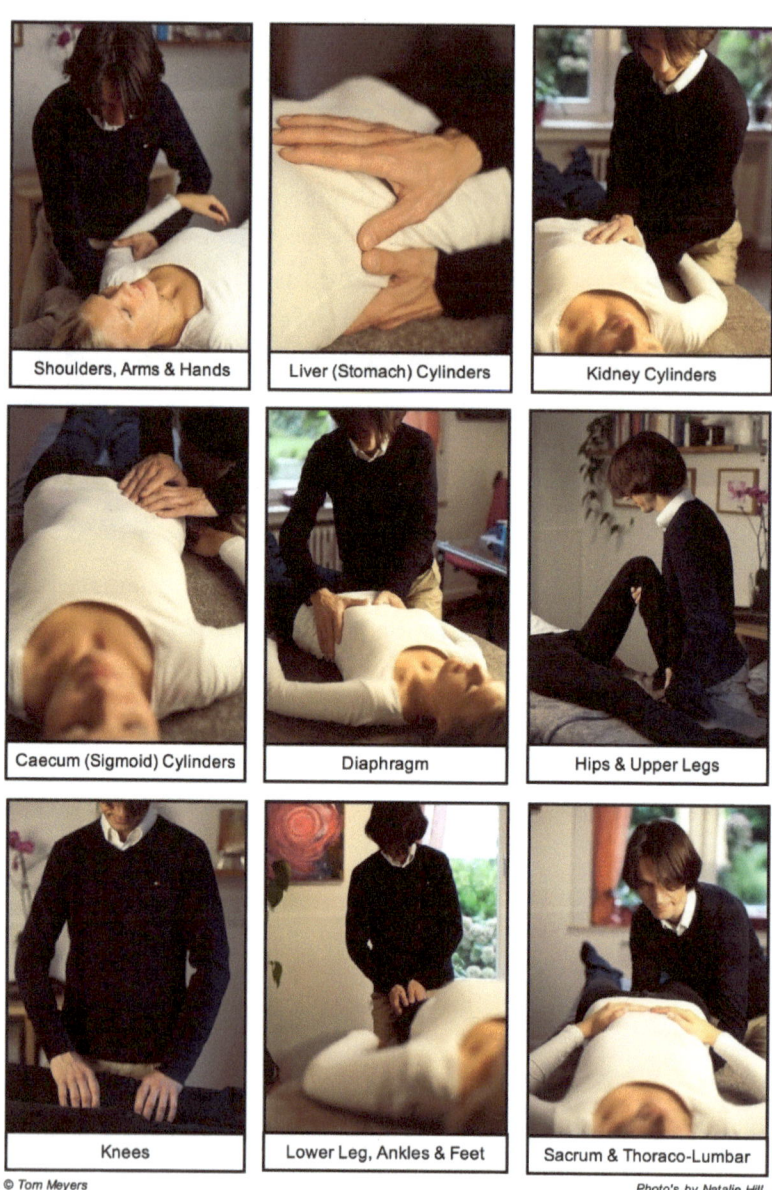

Photo's by Natalie Hill

Figure 2: Reaset Approach hand modalities on the body

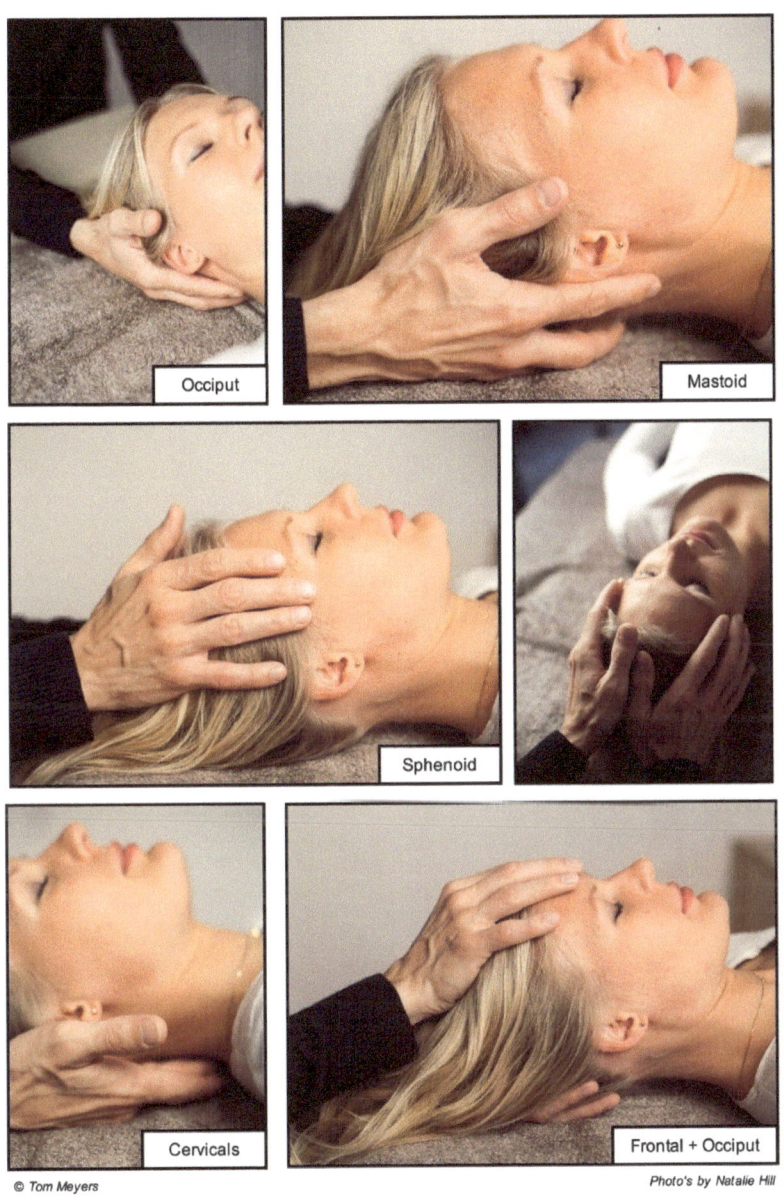

Photo's by Natalie Hill

Figure 3: Reaset Approach hand modalities on head and neck

4.6 STUDY FLOW

This pilot study took place between 13 May 2014 and 20 June 2014 at 'Ostéo & CO' in Brussels, the private practice of the investigator.

Subjects that met all inclusion and exclusion criteria were given an appointment at the private practice of the investigator and sent the informed consent form (ICF) and the STAI Y-2 (t0) in PDF-format by email. This was an amendment to the enrolment (3.1) protocol in the ICF and a preferred means of correspondence by the subjects.

The subjects were asked to return the patient consent form (PCF) and STAI Y-2 by email or at the appointment.

At the appointment:

- Structured pre-treatment interview
- Explanation of the study
- Subjects completed STAI Y-1 (I) and SF-MPQ (I) (t1)
- Subjects washed and dried their hands, removed excessive clothing and lay supine on the treatment table.
- 2 EDA-measuring electrodes were placed on the hypothenar of the non-dominant hand and connected with the MentalBioScreen 'K3' devise.
- HRV-measuring electrodes were placed: One electrode was placed on the right intercostal space 2, parasternal and the second electrode on the left intercostal space 5, medioclavicular. Both electrodes were then connected with the leads to the Biosign® "HRV-Scanner".

The electrodes stayed on the subject until after the t2 measurement. HRV recordings were only effectuated during 5 minutes at t1 and again for 5 minutes at t2, while EDA was recorded continuously from the time the electrodes were placed and the device switched on. To define the start of the t1 and t2, 5-minute EDA recording the investigator pressed the alarm-stamp indicator on the device at the appropriate time. The 5-minute t1 and t2 recordings were then subtracted and analyzed by the software provided with the device.

- 5-minute rest period
- 5-minute baseline of HRV and EDA (t1)
- 25-minute intervention
- 5-minute baseline of HRV and EDA (t2)
- Removal of the electrodes
- Subjects completed STAI Y-1 (II) and SF-MPQ (II) (t2)

The investigator stayed in the room seated behind a desk during the completion of the questionnaires and the 5-minute rest and t1 and t2 measurement period.

Follow-up procedures were explained before the subjects left the practice. This included the follow-up SF-MPQ and the STAI Y-2 respectively scheduled to be received by the subject by email 3 (t3) and 21 (t4) days after the intervention.

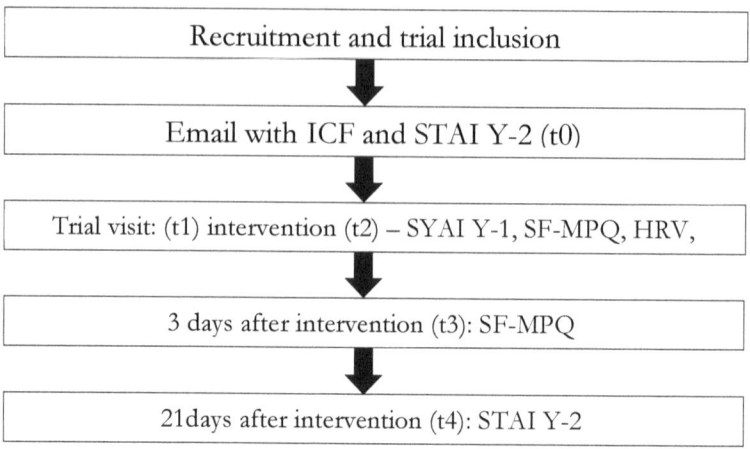

Figure 4: Flow chart from recruitment till end of study

4.7 STATISTICS

The data results are based on 15 subjects divided into 3 groups of 5. Short-term HRV analysis was conducted by the software provided with the Biosign® "HRV-Scanner". EDA analysis was conducted by the software provided with the MentalBioScreen 'K3'. State and Trait anxiety data acquired with the STAY Y-1 and Y-2 were scored for pre to post score differences with the State-Trait Anxiety Inventory for adults scoring key provided by the company Mind Garden Inc. Perceived musculoskeletal pain was scored with the instructions provided by Professor Melzack by email on 21 January 2014 (Add. 9.5). All data were collected and entered in Microsoft Excel for Mac 2011 v.14.4.4 and summarized using descriptive statistics.

5 RESULTS

The 'Reaset Approach' has a measurable influence on the autonomic nervous system, state and trait anxiety and perceived musculoskeletal pain in all three groups. Greater improvements were assessed in the groups which included the intervention on head and neck compared to the body-only group.

5.1 ANS: HEART RATE VARIABILITY

HRV parameters included in this pilot study were: SDNN, SD1 and SD2.

5.1.1 SDNN

In group 'B', the SDNN value increased in 4 out of 5 subjects (t2-t1). Minimum increase was measured in subject 1, which went from 36,61 ± 8,13 to 37,74 ± 10,99 - a difference of 1.13 ms. Maximum increase was measured in subject 6, which went from 43,55 ± 8,13 to 54,2 ± 10,99 - a difference of 10,65 ms. (Fig. 5 and Tbl. 4)

The SDNN value in subject 13 fell from 49,46 ± 8,13 to 28,27 ± 10,99 - a difference of -21,19 ms. (Fig. 5 and Tbl. 4)

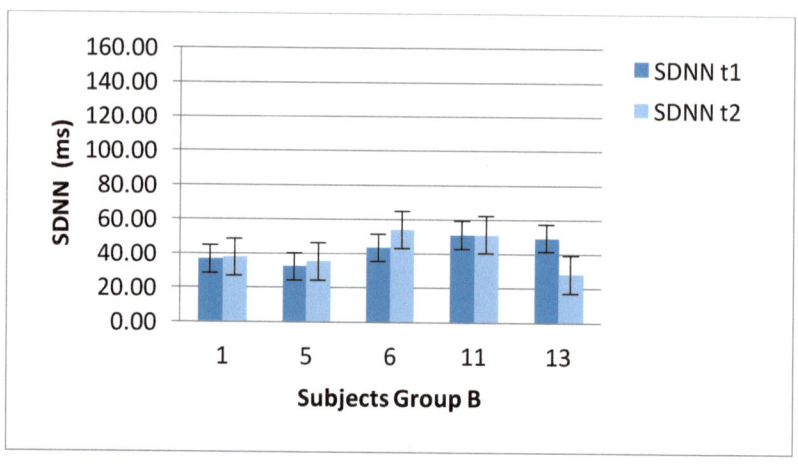

Figure 5: SDNN in group B
Results (ms) before (t1) and after (t2) the intervention by subject

Table 4: SDNN in group B
Results (ms) before (t1) and after (t2) the intervention and difference (t2-t1) by subject

ID	Group	SDNN t1	SDNN t2	SDNN (t2-t1)
1	B	36,61	37,74	1,13
5	B	32,28	35,37	3,09
6	B	43,55	54,2	10,65
11	B	51,22	51,27	0,05
13	B	49,46	28,27	-21,19
Mean		*42,62*	*41,37*	*-1,25*
SD		*8,13*	*10,99*	*11,89*

In group 'HN', the SDNN value increased in 4 out of 5 subjects (t2-t1). Minimum increase was measured in subject 12, which went from 29,76 ± 13,38 to 29,91 ± 35,58 - a difference of 0,15 ms. Maximum increase was measured in subject 3, which went from 56,33 ± 13,38 to 110,94 ± 35,58 - a difference of 54,61 ms. (Fig. 6 and Tbl. 5)

The SDNN value in subject 15 reduced from 33,32 ± 13,38 to 32,08 ± 35,58 a difference of -1,24 ms. (Fig. 6 and Tbl. 5)

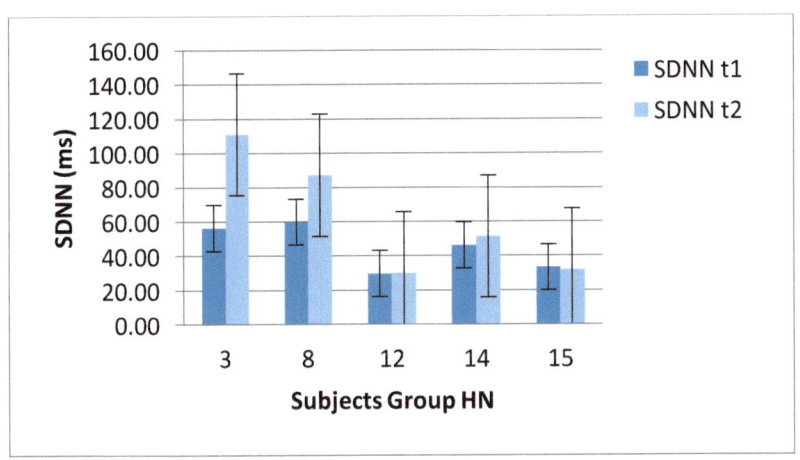

Figure 6: SDNN in group HN
Results (ms) before (t1) and after (t2) the intervention by subject

Table 5: SDNN in group HN
Results (ms) before (t1) and after (t2) the intervention and difference (t2-t1) by subject

ID	Group	SDNN t1	SDNN t2	SDNN (t2-t1)
3	HN	56,33	110,94	54,61
8	HN	59,75	87,15	27,4
12	HN	29,76	29,91	0,15
14	HN	46,19	51,46	5,27
15	HN	33,32	32,08	-1,24
Mean		*45,07*	*62,31*	*17,24*
SD		*13,38*	*35,58*	*23,86*

In group 'HNB', the SDNN value increased in all 5 subjects (t2-t1). Minimum increase was measured in subject 7, which went from 35,8 ± 5,5 to 41,85 ± 8,79 - a difference of 6,05 ms. Maximum increase was measured in subject 4, which went from 36,62 ± 5,5 to 65,93 ± 8,79 - a difference of 29,31 ms. (Fig. 7 and Tbl. 6)

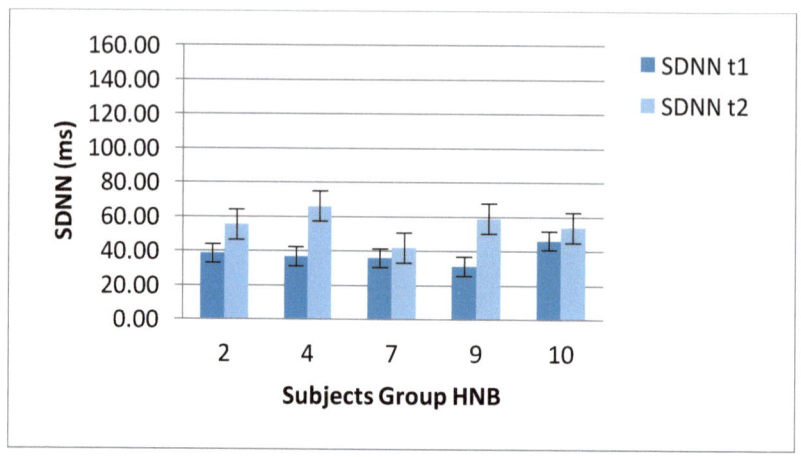

Figure 7: SDNN in group HNB

Results (ms) before (t1) and after (t2) the intervention by subject

Table 6: SDNN in group HNB

Results (ms) before (t1) and after (t2) the intervention and difference (t2-t1) by subject

ID	Group	SDNN t1	SDNN t2	SDNN (t2-t1)
2	HNB	38,36	55,24	16,88
4	HNB	36,62	65,93	29,31
7	HNB	35,80	41,85	6,05
9	HNB	31,02	58,93	27,91
10	HNB	46,15	53,77	7,62
Mean		*37,59*	*55,14*	*17,55*
SD		*5,50*	*8,79*	*10,92*

5.1.2 SD1

In group 'B', the SD1 value increased in 4 out of 5 subjects (t2-t1). Minimum increase was measured in subject 5, which went from 18,01 ± 2,84 to 18,38 ± 7,95 - a difference of 0,37 ms. Maximum increase was measured in subject 6, which went from 24,03 ± 2,84 to 34,94 ± 7,95 - a difference of 10,91 ms. (Fig. 8 and Tbl. 7)

The SD1 value in subject 13 fell from 21,29 ± 2,84 to 15,63 ± 7,95 - a difference of -5,66 ms. (Fig. 8 and Tbl. 7)

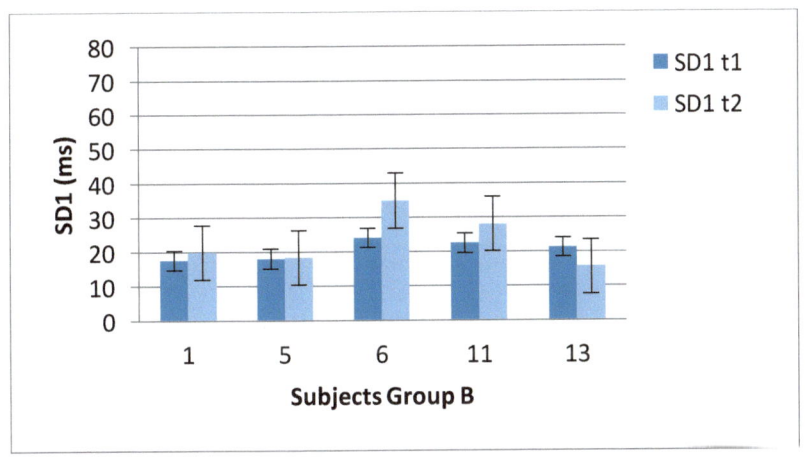

Figure 8: SD1 in group B

Results (ms) before (t1) and after (t2) the intervention by subject

Table 7: SD1 in group B

Results (ms) before (t1) and after (t2) the intervention and difference (t2-t1) by subject

ID	Group	SD1 t1	SD1 t2	SD1 (t2-t1)
1	B	17,51	19,89	2,38
5	B	18,01	18,38	0,37
6	B	24,03	34,94	10,91
11	B	22,52	28,09	5,57
13	B	21,29	15,63	-5,66
Mean		*20,67*	*23,39*	*2,71*
SD		*2,84*	*7,95*	*6,15*

In group 'HN', the SD1 value increased in 3 out of 5 subjects (t2-t1). Minimum increase was measured in subject 8, which went from 46,94 ± 16,83 to 49,61 ± 19,6 - a difference of 2,67 ms. Maximum increase was measured in subject 3, which went from 49,74 ± 16,83 to 58,35 ± 19,6 - a difference of 8,61 ms. (Fig. 9 and Tbl. 8)

The SD1 value in subjects 12 and 14 fell. For subject 12 the SD1 value fell from 13,01 ± 16,83 to 11,79 ± 19,6 - a difference of -1,22 ms. For subject 14 the SD1 value fell from 24,84 ± 16,83 to 23,47 ± 19,6 - a difference of -1,37 ms. (Fig. 9 and Tbl. 8)

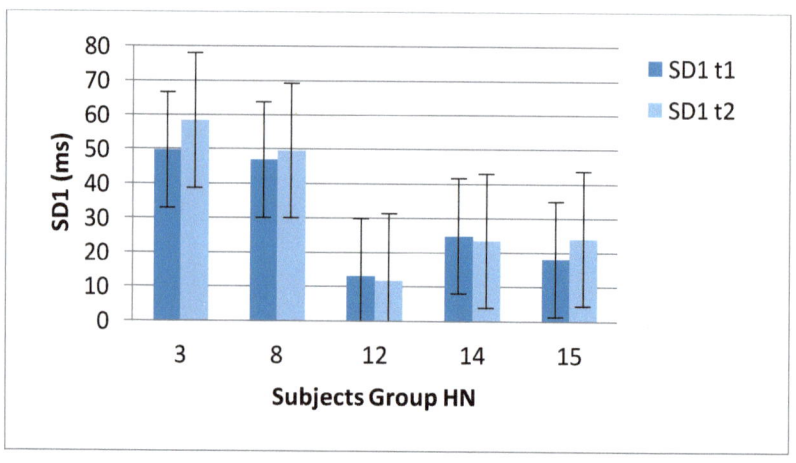

Figure 9: SD1 in group HN

Results (ms) before (t1) and after (t2) the intervention by subject

Table 8: SD1 in group HN

Results (ms) before (t1) and after (t2) the intervention and difference (t2-t1) by subject

ID	Group	SD1 t1	SD1 t2	SD1 (t2-t1)
3	HN	49,74	58,35	8,61
8	HN	46,94	49,61	2,67
12	HN	13,01	11,79	-1,22
14	HN	24,84	23,47	-1,37
15	HN	18,05	24,13	6,08
Mean		30,52	33,47	2,95
SD		16,83	19,60	4,41

In group 'HNB', the SD1 value increased in all 5 subjects (t2-t1). Minimum increase was measured in subject 7, which went from 19,81 ± 6,61 to 21,62 ± 7,08 - a difference of 1,81 ms. Maximum increase was measured in subject 4, which went from 21,34 ± 6,61 to 32,32 ± 7,08 - a difference of 10,98 ms. (Fig. 10 and Tbl. 9)

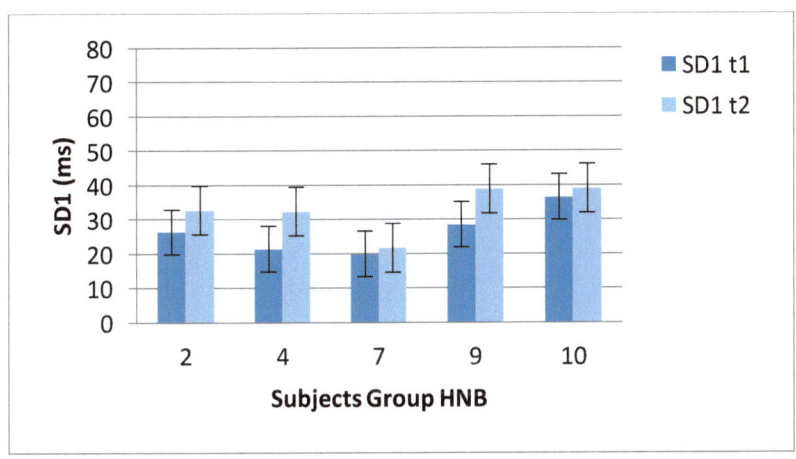

Figure 10: SD1 in group HNB

Results (ms) before (t1) and after (t2) the intervention by subject

Table 9: SD1 in group HNB

Results (ms) before (t1) and after (t2) the intervention and difference (t2-t1) by subject

ID	Group	SD1 t1	SD1 t2	SD1 (t2-t1)
2	HNB	26,33	32,71	6,38
4	HNB	21,34	32,32	10,98
7	HNB	19,81	21,62	1,81
9	HNB	28,42	38,88	10,46
10	HNB	36,48	38,98	2,5
Mean		*26,48*	*32,90*	*6,43*
SD		*6,61*	*7,08*	*4,29*

5.1.3 SD2

In group 'B', the SD2 value increased in 3 out of 5 subjects (t2-t1). Minimum increase was measured in subject 1, which went from 48,73 ± 11,48 to 49,53 ± 13,59 - a difference of 0,8 ms. Maximum increase was measured in subject 6, which went from 56,71 ± 11,48 to 68,22 ± 13,59 - a difference of 11,51 ms. (Fig. 11 and Tbl. 10)

The SD2 value in subjects 11 and 13 fell. For subject 11 the SD2 value fell from 68,84 ± 11,48 to 66,85 ± 13,59 - a difference of -1,99 ms. For subject 13 the SD2 value fell from 66,63 ± 11,48 to 36,79 ± 13,59 - a difference of -29,84 ms. (Fig. 11 and Tbl. 10)

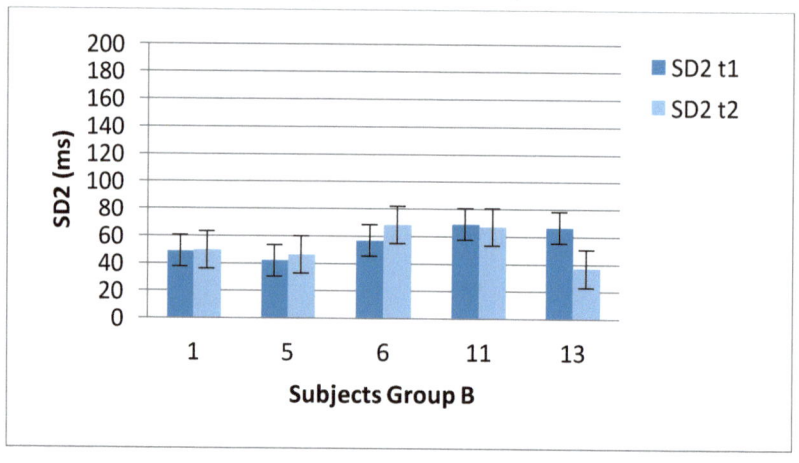

Figure 11: SD2 in group B

Results (ms) before (t1) and after (t2) the intervention by subject

Table 10: SD2 in group B

Results (ms) before (t1) and after (t2) the intervention and difference (t2-t1) by subject

ID	Group	SD2 t1	SD2 t2	SD2 (t2-t1)
1	B	48,73	49,53	0,8
5	B	41,95	46,52	4,57
6	B	56,71	68,22	11,51
11	B	68,84	66,85	-1,99
13	B	66,63	36,79	-29,84
Mean		*56,57*	*53,58*	*-2,99*
SD		*11,48*	*13,59*	*15,84*

In group 'HN', the SD2 value increased in 4 out of 5 subjects (t2-t1). Minimum increase was measured in subject 12, which went from 40,03 ± 12,94 to 40,63 ± 46,86 - a difference of 0,6 ms. Maximum increase was measured in subject 3, which went from 62,22 ± 12,94 to 145,64 ± 46,86 - a difference of 83,42 ms. (Fig. 12 and Tbl. 11)

The SD2 value in subject 15 fell from 43,53 ± 12,94 to 38,41 ± 46,86 - a difference of -5,12 ms. (Fig. 12 and Tbl. 11)

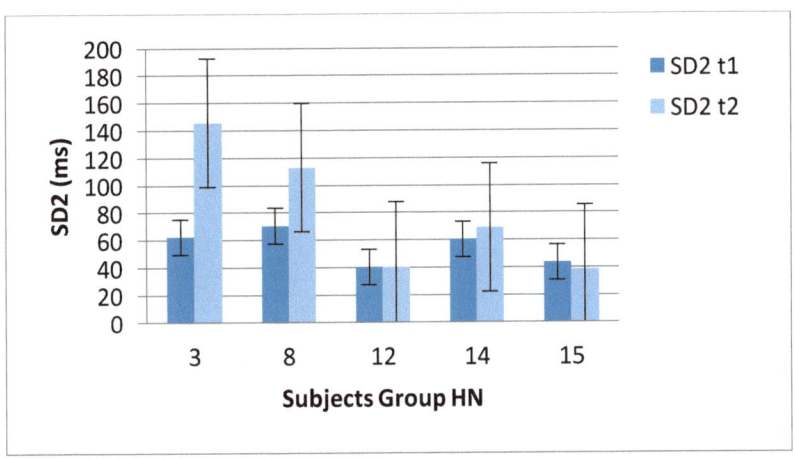

Figure 12: SD2 in group HN
Results (ms) before (t1) and after (t2) the intervention by subject

Table 11: SD2 in group HN
Results (ms) before (t1) and after (t2) the intervention and difference (t2-t1) by subject

ID	Group	SD2 t1	SD2 t2	SD2 (t2-t1)
3	HN	62,22	145,64	83,42
8	HN	70,26	112,83	42,57
12	HN	40,03	40,63	0,6
14	HN	60,41	68,88	8,47
15	HN	43,53	38,41	-5,12
Mean		*55,29*	*81,28*	*25,99*
SD		*12,94*	*46,86*	*37,06*

In group 'HNB', the SD2 value increased in all 5 subjects (t2-t1). Minimum increase was measured in subject 7, which went from 46,59 ± 7,54 to 55,1 ± 11,85 - a difference of 8,51 ms. Maximum increase was measured in subject 9, which went from 33,43 ± 7,54 to 73,72 ± 11,85 - a difference of 40,29 ms. (Fig. 13 and Tbl. 12)

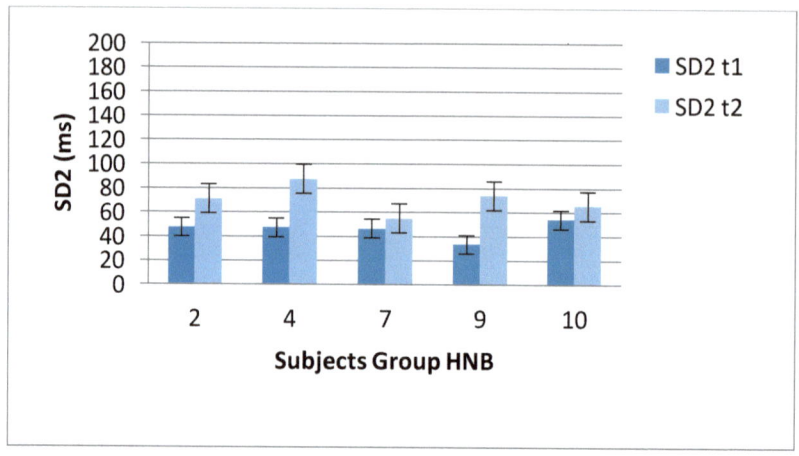

Figure 13: SD2 in group HNB

Results (ms) before (t1) and after (t2) the intervention by subject

Table 12: SD2 in group HNB

Results (ms) before (t1) and after (t2) the intervention and difference (t2-t1) by subject

ID	Group	SD2 t1	SD2 t2	SD2 (t2-t1)
2	HNB	47,44	70,94	23,5
4	HNB	47,18	87,45	40,27
7	HNB	46,59	55,1	8,51
9	HNB	33,43	73,72	40,29
10	HNB	54,12	65,3	11,18
Mean		*45,75*	*70,50*	*24,75*
SD		*7,54*	*11,85*	*15,26*

5.2 ANS: ELECTRO-DERMAL ACTIVITY

In group 'B', the EDA fell in 2 out of 5 subjects (t2-t1). Minimum reduction was measured in subject 11, which went from $0,9 \pm 0,54$ to $0,8 \pm 1,71$ - a difference of -0,1 µS. Maximum reduction was measured in subject 1, which went from $0,9 \pm 0,54$ to $0,7 \pm 1,71$ - a difference of -0,2 µS. (Fig. 14 and Tbl. 13)

The EDA for subjects 5, 6 and 13 increased. For subject 5 the increase was from $2,0 \pm 0,54$ to $4,9 \pm 1,71$, a difference of 2,9 µS. For subject 6 the increase was from $1,2 \pm 0,54$ to $2,5 \pm 1,71$ - a difference of 1,3 µS. For subject 13 the increase was from $1,9 \pm 0,54$ to $2,6 \pm 1,71$ - a difference of 0,7 µS. (Fig. 14 and Tbl. 13)

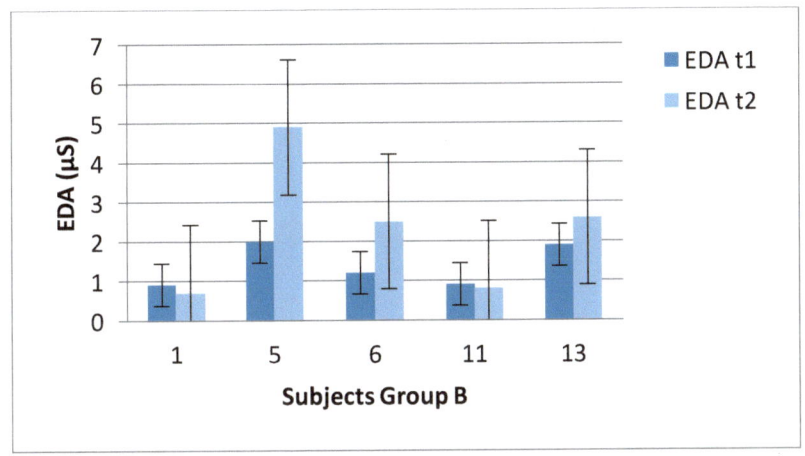

Figure 14: EDA in group B

Results (µS) before (t1) and after (t2) the intervention by subject

Table 13: EDA in group B

Results (µS) before (t1) and after (t2) the intervention and difference (t2-t1) by subject

ID	Group	EDA t1	EDA t2	EDA (t2-t1)
1	B	0,9	0,7	-0,20
5	B	2	4,9	2,90
6	B	1,2	2,5	1,30
11	B	0,9	0,8	-0,10
13	B	1,9	2,6	0,70
Mean		*1,38*	*2,30*	*0,92*
SD		*0,54*	*1,71*	*1,27*

In group 'HN', the EDA fell in 4 subjects (t2-t1). For subject 3 no
EDA registration was recorded for reasons unknown to the
investigator. Minimum reduction was measured in subject 8, which
went from 1,3 ± 0,46 to 1,1 ± 0,3 - a difference of -0,2 µS. Maximum
reduction was measured in subject 12, which went from 2,4 ± 0,46 to
1,7 ± 0,3 - a difference of -0,7 µS. (Fig. 15 and Tbl. 14)

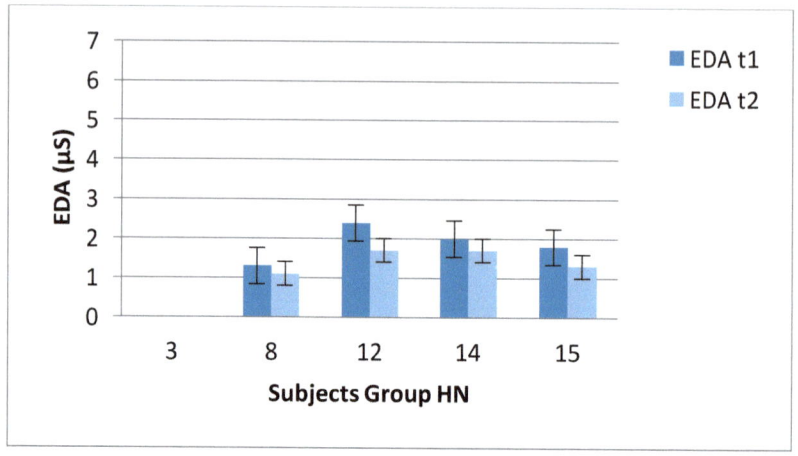

Figure 15: EDA in group HN

Results (µS) before (t1) and after (t2) the intervention by subject.*

Table 14: EDA in group HN

Results (µS) before (t1) and after (t2) the intervention and difference
(t2-t1) by subject *

ID	Group	EDA t1	EDA t2	EDA (t2-t1)
3	HN			
8	HN	1,3	1,1	-0,20
12	HN	2,4	1,7	-0,70
14	HN	2	1,7	-0,30
15	HN	1,8	1,3	-0,50
Mean		*1,88*	*1,45*	*-0,43*
SD		*0,46*	*0,30*	*0,22*

* Subject 3 had erroneous EDA measurements

In group 'HNB', the EDA fell in 4 out of 5 subjects (t2-t1). Minimum reduction was measured in subject 7, which went from 0,9 ± 0,8 to 0,8 ± 1,01 - a difference of -0,1 μS. Maximum reduction was measured in subject 4, which went from 2,8 ± 0,8 to 2,3 ± 1,01 - a difference of -0,5 μS. (Fig. 16 and Tbl. 15)

The EDA for subject 10 increased from 2,5 ± 0,8 to 3,3 ± 1,01 a difference of 0,8 μS.

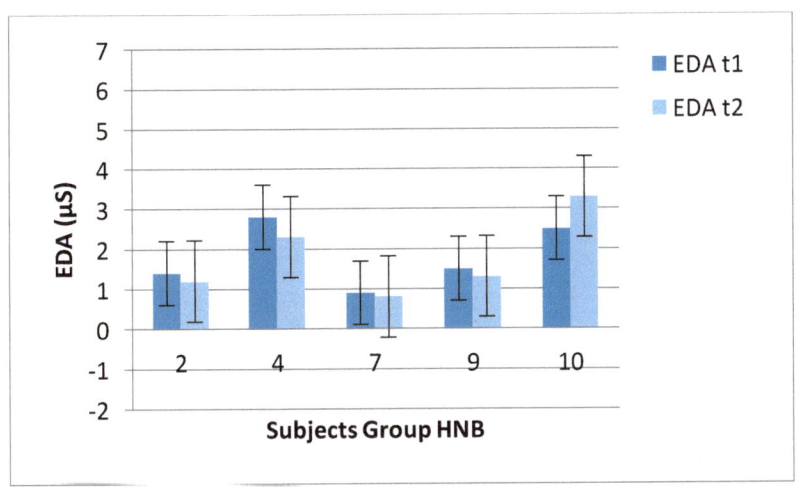

Figure 16: EDA in group HNB

Results (μS) before (t1) and after (t2) the intervention by subject

Table 15: EDA in group HNB

Results (μS) before (t1) and after (t2) the intervention and difference (t2-t1) by subject

ID	Group	EDA t1	EDA t2	EDA (t2-t1)
2	HNB	1,4	1,2	-0,20
4	HNB	2,8	2,3	-0,50
7	HNB	0,9	0,8	-0,10
9	HNB	1,5	1,3	-0,20
10	HNB	2,5	3,3	0,80
Mean		*1,82*	*1,78*	*-0,04*
SD		*0,80*	*1,01*	*0,49*

5.3 ANXIETY

State and trait anxiety was measured with the State Trait Anxiety Inventory (STAI). Form STAI Y-1 was used for state anxiety and form STAI Y-2 for trait anxiety. The scores range from minimum 20 to maximum score 80, with higher scores positively correlating with higher anxiety.

5.3.1 STATE ANXIETY

In group 'B', state anxiety was reduced in all 5 subjects (t2-t1). Minimum reduction was measured in subjects 1 and 6. Subject 1 went from 26 ± 7,12 to 22 ± 4,09 and subject 6 went from 35 ± 7,12 to 31 ± 4,09, the difference for both being -4. Maximum reduction was measured in subject 13, which went from 44 ± 7,12 to 26 ± 4,09 - a difference of -18. (Fig. 17 and Tbl. 16)

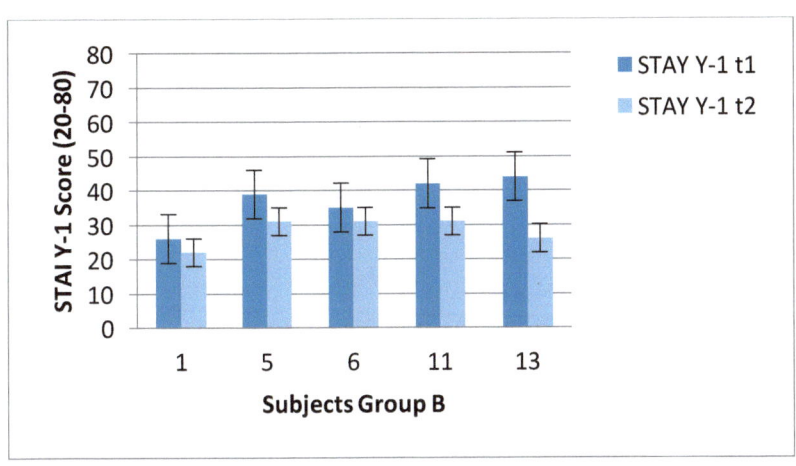

Figure 17: STAI Y-1 in group B

Results (score 20-80) before (t1) and after (t2) the intervention by subject

Table 16: STAI Y-1 in group B

Results (score 20-80) before (t1) and after (t2) the intervention and difference (t2-t1) by subject

ID	Group	STAY Y-1 t1	STAY Y-1 t2	STAY Y-1 (t2-t1)
1	B	26	22	-4
5	B	39	31	-8
6	B	35	31	-4
11	B	42	31	-11
13	B	44	26	-18
Mean		*37,20*	*28,20*	*-9,00*
SD		*7,12*	*4,09*	*5,83*

In group 'HN', state anxiety was reduced in all 5 subjects (t2-t1). Minimum reduction was measured in subject 12, which went from 25 ± 7,31 to 20 ± 2,88 - a difference of -5. Maximum reduction was measured in subject 14, which went from 42 ± 7,31 to 20 ± 2,88 - a difference of -22. Subjects 14 and 15 went down to the minimum score of 20. (Fig. 18 and Tbl. 17)

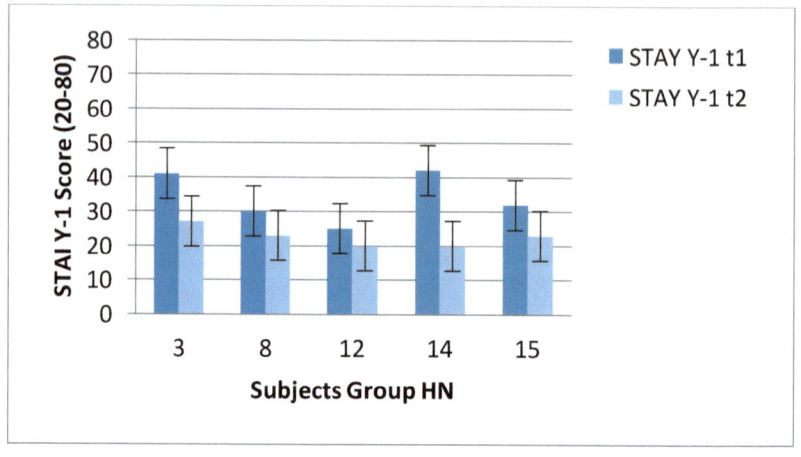

Figure 18: STAI Y-1 in group HN

Results (score 20-80) before (t1) and after (t2) the intervention by subject

Table 17: STAI Y-1 in group HN

Results (score 20-80) before (t1) and after (t2) the intervention and difference (t2-t1) by subject

ID	Group	STAY Y-1 t1	STAY Y-1 t2	STAY Y-1 (t2-t1)
3	HN	41	27	-14
8	HN	30	23	-7
12	HN	25	20	-5
14	HN	42	20	-22
15	HN	32	23	-9
Mean		*34,00*	*22,60*	*-11,40*
SD		*7,31*	*2,88*	*6,80*

In group 'HNB', state anxiety was reduced in all 5 subjects (t2-t1). Minimum reduction was measured in subject 10, which went from 36 ± 8,41 to 29 ± 7,5 - a difference of -7. Maximum reduction was measured in subject 7, which went from 54 ± 8,41 to 42 ± 7,5 - a difference of -12. (Fig. 19 and Tbl. 18)

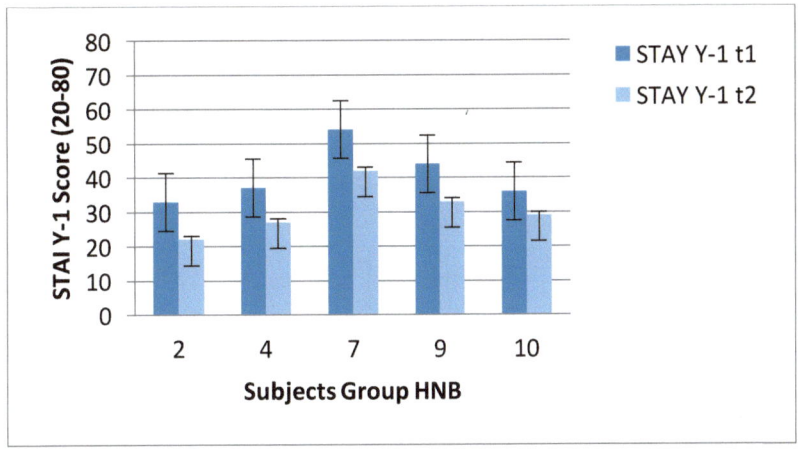

Figure 19: STAI Y-1 in group HNB

Results (score 20-80) before (t1) and after (t2) the intervention by subject

Table 18: STAI Y-1 in group HNB

Results (score 20-80) before (t1) and after (t2) the intervention and difference (t2-t1) by subject

ID	Group	STAY Y-1 t1	STAY Y-1 t2	STAY Y-1 (t2-t1)
2	HNB	33	22	-11
4	HNB	37	27	-10
7	HNB	54	42	-12
9	HNB	44	33	-11
10	HNB	36	29	-7
Mean		*40,80*	*30,60*	*-10,20*
SD		*8,41*	*7,50*	*1,92*

5.3.2 TRAIT ANXIETY

In group 'B', trait anxiety was reduced in all 5 subjects (t4-t0). Minimum reduction was measured in subject 13, which went from 35 ± 7,36 to 30 ± 7,27 - a difference of -5.

Maximum reduction was measured in subject 5, which went from 44 ± 7,36 to 31 ± 7,27 - a difference of -13. (Fig. 20 and Tbl. 19)

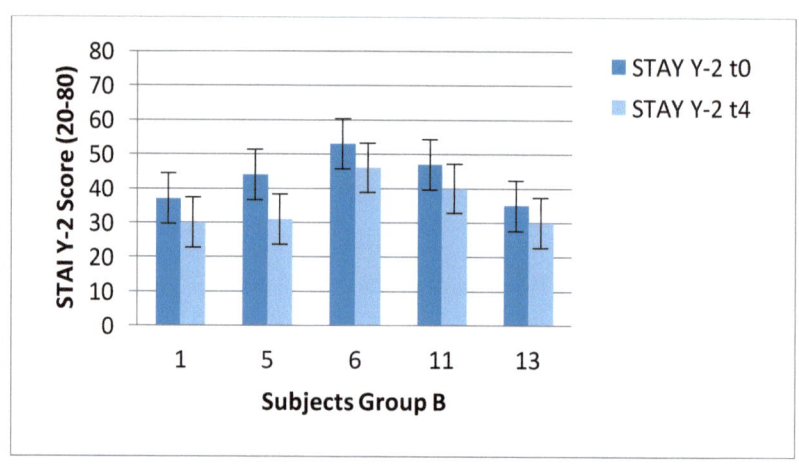

Figure 20: STAI Y-2 in group B

Results (20-80) prior the appointment (t0) and 21-days after (t4) the intervention by subject

Table 19: STAI Y-2 in group B

Results (20-80) prior the appointment (t0) and 21-days after (t4) the intervention and the difference (t4-t0) by subject

ID	Group	STAY Y-2 t0	STAY Y-2 t4	STAY Y-2 (t4-t0)
1	B	37	30	-7
5	B	44	31	-13
6	B	53	46	-7
11	B	47	40	-7
13	B	35	30	-5
Mean		*43,20*	*35,40*	*-7,80*
SD		*7,36*	*7,27*	*3,03*

In group 'HN', trait anxiety was reduced in all 5 subjects (t4-t0). Minimum reduction was measured in subject 14, which went from 33 ± 7,13 to 31 ± 7,02 - a difference of -2.

Maximum reduction was measured in subject 15, which went from 41 ± 7,13 to 27 ± 7,02 - a difference of -14. (Fig. 21 and Tbl. 20)

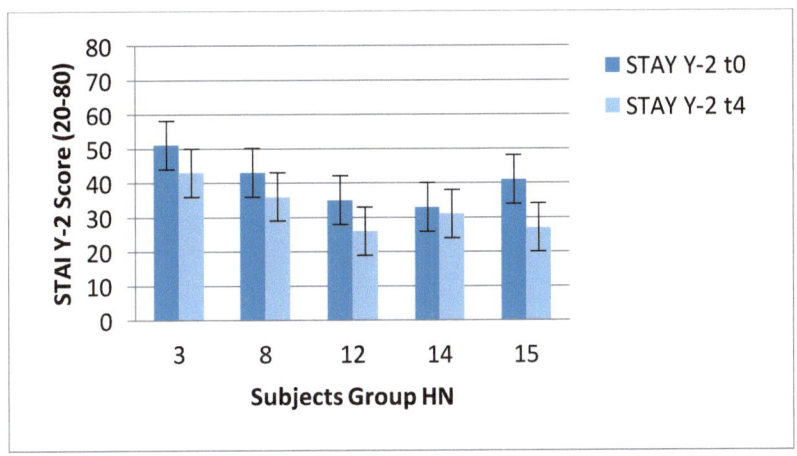

Figure 21: STAI Y-2 in group HN

Results (20-80) prior the appointment (t0) and 21-days after (t4) the intervention by subject

Table 20: STAI Y-2 in group HN

Results (20-80) prior the appointment (t0) and 21-days after (t4) the intervention and the difference (t4-t0) by subject

ID	Group	STAY Y-2 t0	STAY Y-2 t4	STAY Y-2 (t4-t0)
3	HN	51	43	-8
8	HN	43	36	-7
12	HN	35	26	-9
14	HN	33	31	-2
15	HN	41	27	-14
Mean		*40,60*	*32,60*	*-8,00*
SD		*7,13*	*7,02*	*4,30*

In group 'HNB', trait anxiety was reduced in 3 out of 5 subjects (t4-t0). Minimum reduction was measured in subject 2, which reduced from 45 ± 5,77 to 44 ± 2,41 - a difference of -1.

Maximum reduction was measured in subject 7, which went from 56 ± 5,77 to 48 ± 2,41 - a difference of -8. Subject 4 remained unchanged. (Fig. 22 and Tbl. 21)

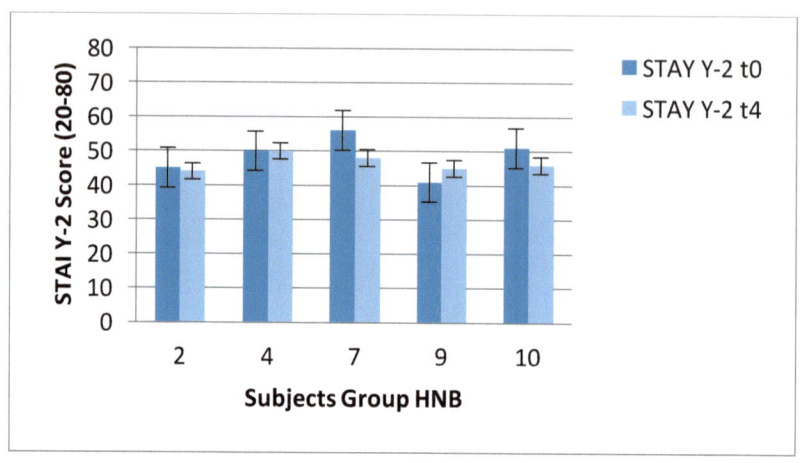

Figure 22: STAI Y-2 in group HNB

Results (20-80) prior the appointment (t0) and 21-days after (t4) the intervention by subject

Table 21: STAI Y-2 in group HNB

Results (20-80) prior the appointment (t0) and 21-days after (t4) the intervention and the difference (t4-t0) by subject

ID	Group	STAY Y-2 t0	STAY Y-2 t4	STAY Y-2 (t4-t0)
2	HNB	45	44	-1
4	HNB	50	50	0
7	HNB	56	48	-8
9	HNB	41	45	4
10	HNB	51	46	-5
Mean		48,60	46,60	-2,00
SD		5,77	2,41	4,64

5.4 MUSCULOSKELETAL PAIN

Musculoskeletal pain was measured immediately before (t1), right after (t2) and 3 days after (t3) the intervention with the SF-MPQ and is represented by a VAS scale and a total SF-MPQ (Present Pain Intensity) score (T=S+A+E).

5.4.1 VISUAL ANALOGUE SCALE

In group 'B', VAS score between t1 and t2 (t2-t1) was reduced in 4 out of 5 subjects. Minimum reduction was measured in subject 5, which went from 24 ± 18,35 to 13 ± 16,82 a difference of -11 mm. Maximum reduction was measured in subject 13, which went from 68 ± 18,35 to 12 ± 16,82 - a difference of -56 mm.

VAS score at t3 compared to t1 (t3-t1) was reduced in 4 subjects. No scores were registered for subject 13 at t3 as the subject failed to return the SF-MPQ t3. Minimum reduction was measured in subject 11, which went from 25 ± 18,35 to 24 ± 10,42 - a difference of -1 mm. Maximum reduction was measured in subject 1, which went from 49 ± 18,35 to 0 ± 10,42 - a difference of -49 mm. (Fig. 23 and Tbl. 22)

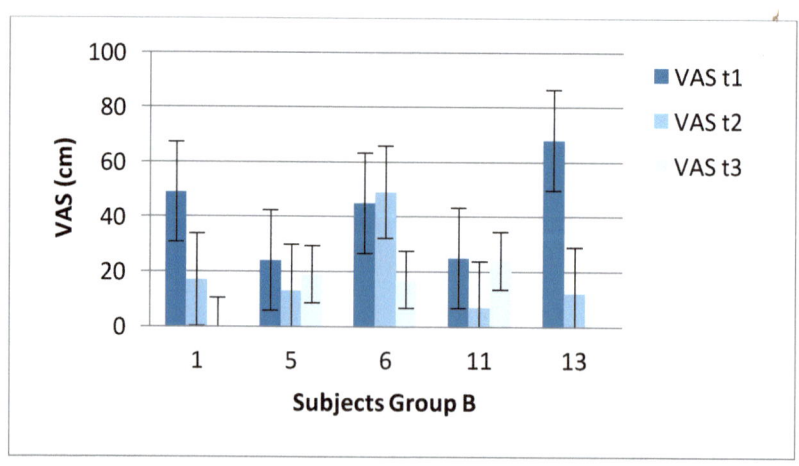

Figure 23: VAS in group B

Results (mm) before (t1), after (t2) and 3 days after (t3) the intervention by subject

Table 22: VAS in group B

Results (mm) before (t1) and after (t2) and 3 days after (t3) the intervention and difference between t1 and t2 (t2-t1) and t1 and t3 (t3-t1) by subject

ID	Group	VAS t1	VAS t2	VAS (t2-t1)	VAS t3	VAS (t3-t2)	VAS (t3-t1)
1	B	49	17	-32	0	-17	-49
5	B	24	13	-11	19	6	-5
6	B	45	49	4	17	-32	-28
11	B	25	7	-18	24	17	-1
13	B	68	12	-56			
Mean		42,20	19,60	-22,60	15,00	-6,50	-20,75
SD		18,35	16,82	22,73	10,42	22,13	22,28

In group 'HN', VAS score between t1 and t2 (t2-t1) was reduced in all 5 subjects. Minimum reduction was measured in subject 15, which went from 8 ± 24,21 to 0 ± 26,4 - a difference of -8 mm. Maximum reduction was measured in subject 14, which went from 48 ± 24,21 to 0 ± 26,4 - a difference of -48 mm. Subjects 14 and 15 perceived pain reduced to no pain.

VAS score at t3 compared to t1 (t3-t1) was reduced in all 5 subjects. Minimum reduction was measured in subject 15, which went from 8 ± 24,21 to 0 ± 26,4 - a difference of -8 mm thus staying at no pain compared to t2. Maximum reduction was measured in subject 8, which went from 60 ± 24,21 to 13 ± 26,48 - a difference of -47. In subject 3 the VAS score fell from 41 ± 24,21 to 0 ± 26,48 - a difference of -41 mm. (Fig. 24 and Tbl. 23)

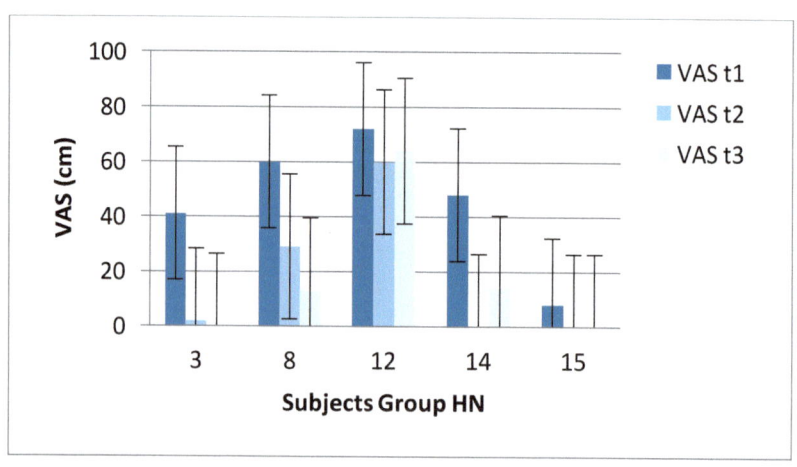

Figure 24: VAS in group HN
Results (mm) before (t1), after (t2) and 3 days after (t3) the intervention by subject

Table 23: VAS in group HN

Results (mm) before (t1) and after (t2) and 3 days after (t3) the
intervention and difference between t1 and t2 (t2-t1) and t1 and t3
(t3-t1) by subject

ID	Group	VAS t1	VAS t2	VAS (t2-t1)	VAS t3	VAS (t3-t2)	VAS (t3-t1)
3	HN	41	2	-39	0	-2	-41
8	HN	60	29	-31	13	-16	-47
12	HN	72	60	-12	64	4	-8
14	HN	48	0	-48	14	14	-34
15	HN	8	0	-8	0	0	-8
Mean		45,80	18,20	-27,60	18,20	0,00	-27,60
SD		24,21	26,40	17,21	26,48	10,86	18,47

In group 'HNB', VAS score between t1 and t2 (t2-t1) was reduced in all 5 subjects. Minimum reduction was measured in subject 10, which went from 31 ± 13,27 to 23 ± 12,08 - a difference of -8 mm. Maximum reduction was measured in subject 4, which went from 55 ± 13,27 to 23 ± 12,08 - a difference of -32 mm.

VAS score at t3 compared to t1 (t3-t1) was reduced in all 5 subjects. Minimum reduction was measured in subject 9, which went from 31 ± 13,27 to 30 ± 19,46 - a difference of -1 mm. Maximum reduction was measured in subject 2, which went from 54 ± 13,27 to 11 ± 19,46 - a difference of -43 mm. (Fig. 25 and Tbl. 24)

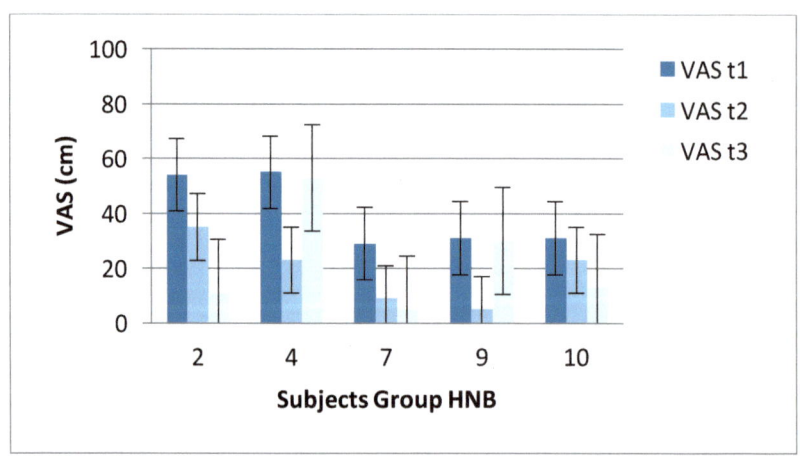

Figure 25: VAS in group HNB
Results (mm) before (t1), after (t2) and 3 days after (t3) the intervention by subject

Table 24: VAS in group HNB

Results (mm) before (t1) and after (t2) and 3 days after (t3) the
intervention and difference between t1 and t2 (t2-t1) and t1 and t3
(t3-t1) by subject

ID	Group	VAS t1	VAS t2	VAS (t2-t1)	VAS t3	VAS (t3-t2)	VAS (t3-t1)
2	HNB	54	35	-19	11	-24	-43
4	HNB	55	23	-32	53	30	-2
7	HNB	29	9	-20	5	-4	-24
9	HNB	31	5	-26	30	25	-1
10	HNB	31	23	-8	13	-10	-18
Mean		*40,00*	*19,00*	*-21,00*	*22,40*	*3,40*	*-17,60*
SD		*13,27*	*12,08*	*8,94*	*19,46*	*23,23*	*17,36*

5.4.2 TOTAL SHORT-FORM MCGILL PAIN QUESTIONNAIRE

In group 'B', total SF-MPQ (Tbl. 28, chapter 9.1) score between t1 and t2 (t2-t1) was reduced in 4 subjects. Minimum reduction was measured in subject 5, which went from 5 ± 2,39 to 2 ± 0,55 - a difference of -3. Maximum reduction was measured in subject 13, which went from 9 ± 2,39 to 2 ± 0,55 - a difference of -7. For subject 6 there was no change in total SF-MPQ between t1 and t2 .

Total SF-MPQ score (Tbl. 28, chapter 9.1) at t3 in comparison with t1 (t3-t) was reduced in 4 subjects. No scores were registered for subject 13 at t3 as the subject failed to return the SF-MPQ t3. Minimum reduction was measured in subjects 5 and 6. Subject 5 went from 5 ± 2,39 to 4 ± 1,91 and subject 6 - for whom the score remained unchanged between t1 and t2 - went from 3 ± 2,39 to 2 ± 1,91 - a difference of -1 in both cases. Maximum reduction was measured in subject 1, which went from 6 ± 2,39 to 0 ± 1,91 - a difference of -6. (Fig. 26 and Tbl. 25)

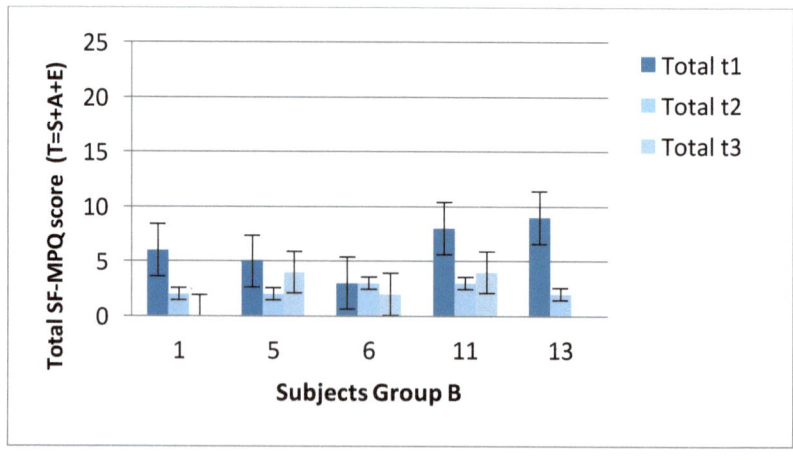

Figure 26: SF-MPQ in group B

Results (T=S+A+E) before (t1), after (t2) and 3 days after (t3) the intervention by subject

Table 25: Total SF-MPQ in group B

Results (T=S+A+E) before (t1), after (t2) and 3 days after (t3) the intervention and difference between t1 and t2 (t2-t1) and t1 and t3 (t3-t1) by subject

ID	Group	Total t1	Total t2	Total (t2-t1)	Total t3	Total (t3-t2)	Total (t3-t1)
1	B	6	2	-4	0	-2	-6
5	B	5	2	-3	4	2	-1
6	B	3	3	0	2	-1	-1
11	B	8	3	-5	4	1	-4
13	B	9	2	-7			
Mean		6,20	2,40	-3,80	2,50	0,00	-3,00
SD		2,39	0,55	2,59	1,91	1,83	2,45

In group 'HN', total SF-MPQ score (Tbl. 28, chapter 9.1) between t1 and t2 (t2-t1) was reduced in 4 subjects. Minimum reduction was measured in subject 15, which went from 3 ± 5,26 to 0 ± 7,43 - a difference of -3. Maximum reduction was measured in subject 3, which went from 8 ± 5,26 to 0 ± 7,43 - a difference of -7. For subjects 3, 14 and 15 total SF-MPQ was reduced to no pain at t2. For subject 6 there was no change in total SF-MPQ between t1 and t2 .

Total SF-MPQ score (Tbl. 28, chapter 9.1) at t3 in comparison with t1 (t3-t) was reduced in all subjects. Minimum reduction was measured in subject 15, which went from 3 ± 5,26 to 2 ± 5,5 - a difference of -1. Maximum reduction was measured in subject 3, which went from 8 ± 5,26 to 0 ± 5,5 - a difference of -8. For subject 3 total SF-MPQ reduced to no pain at t3 (Fig. 27 and Tbl. 26)

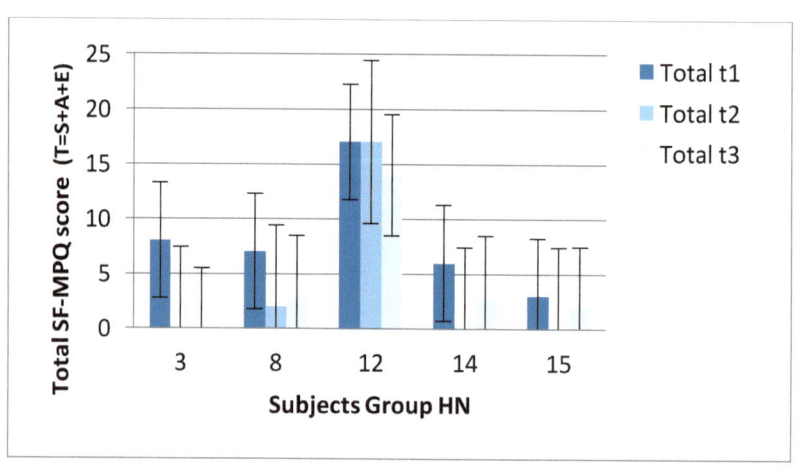

Figure 27: SF-MPQ in group HN
Results (T=S+A+E) before (t1), after (t2) and 3 days after (t3) the intervention by subject

Table 26: Total SF-MPQ in group HN

Results (T=S+A+E) before (t1), after (t2) and 3 days after (t3) the intervention and difference between t1 and t2 (t2-t1) and t1 and t3 (t3-t1) by subject

ID	Group	Total t1	Total t2	Total (t2-t1)	Total t3	Total (t3-t2)	Total (t3-t1)
3	HN	8	0	-8	0	0	-8
8	HN	7	2	-5	3	1	-4
12	HN	17	17	0	14	-3	-3
14	HN	6	0	-6	3	3	-3
15	HN	3	0	-3	2	2	-1
Mean		*8,20*	*3,80*	*-4,40*	*4,40*	*0,60*	*-3,80*
SD		*5,26*	*7,43*	*3,05*	*5,50*	*2,30*	*2,59*

In group 'HNB', total SF-MPQ score (Tbl. 28, chapter 9.1) between t1 and t2 (t2-t1) was reduced in all subjects. Minimum reduction was measured in subjects 2 and 4. Subject 2 went from 8 ± 1,14 to 5 ± 1,95 and subject 4 went from 5 ± 1,14 to 2 ± 1,95 - a difference fof -3 in both cases. Maximum reduction was measured in subject 9, which went from 6 ± 1,14 to 0 ± 1,95 - a difference of -6. For subject 9 total SF-MPQ was reduced to no pain at t2.

Total SF-MPQ score (Tbl. 28, chapter 9.1) at t3 in comparison with t1 (t3-t) was reduced in 4 out of 5 subjects. Minimum reduction was measured in subjects 7,9 and 10. Subjects 6 and 9 went from 6 ± 1,14 to 2 ± 1,22 and subject 10 went from 7 ± 1,14 to 3 ± 1,22 - a difference of -4 in all 3 cases. Maximum reduction was measured in subject 2, which went from 8 ± 2,39 to 3 ± 1,22 - a difference of -5. For subject 7 total SF-MPQ was reduced to no pain at t3. (Fig. 28 and Tbl. 27)

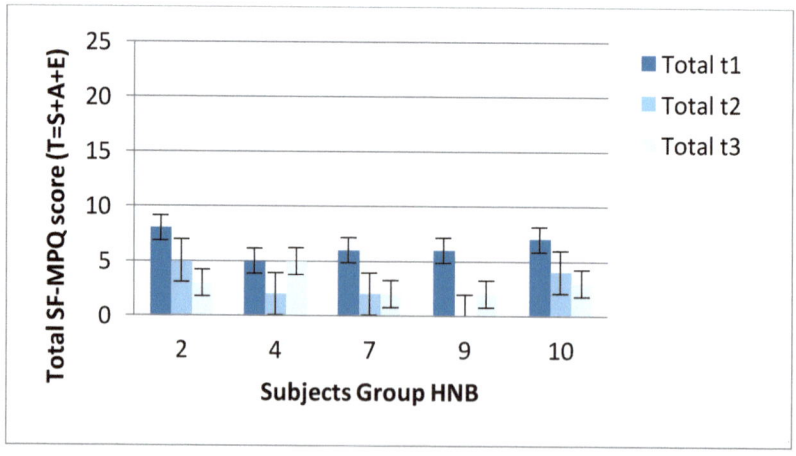

Figure 28: SF-MPQ in group HNB

Results (T=S+A+E) before (t1), after (t2) and 3 days after (t3) the intervention by subject

Table 27: Total SF-MPQ in group HNB

Results (T=S+A+E) before (t1), after (t2) and 3 days after (t3) the intervention and difference between t1 and t2 (t2-t1) and t1 and t3 (t3-t1) by subject

ID	Group	Total t1	Total t2	Total (t2-t1)	Total t3	Total (t3-t2)	Total (t3-t1)
2	HNB	8	5	-3	3	-2	-5
4	HNB	5	2	-3	5	3	0
7	HNB	6	2	-4	2	0	-4
9	HNB	6	0	-6	2	2	-4
10	HNB	7	4	-3	3	-1	-4
Mean		6,40	2,60	-3,80	3,00	0,40	-3,40
SD		1,14	1,95	1,30	1,22	2,07	1,95

6 DISCUSSION

This pilot study tested the feasibility and treatment effect for a randomized controlled trial to evaluate the effect of 3 different interventions (B, HN and HNB), based on the Reaset Approach, on the autonomic nervous system, self-reported state and trait anxiety levels and self-assessed perceived musculoskeletal pain in patients with work-related stress.

6.1 DISCUSSION OF THE METHOD

For this study 42 subjects were recruited over a 1-month period. However, only 15 of these - 13 women and 2 men - met all the eligibility criteria. The main reason for exclusion was insufficient knowledge of the English language (English being the language in which the study was conducted and the questionnaires made up). The study was situated in Brussels, which has a very large English speaking community, but which is predominantly French-speaking. To be able to recruit enough subjects for the follow-up study it is recommended to include a French protocol and questionnaires.

The second most common factor for exclusion was the absence of musculoskeletal pain in subjects. Musculoskeletal pain was an essential inclusion criterion in the study and this should have been made clearer in the recruitment announcements. Priority should also the question 'Do you have muscular tension or pain?' during the structured interview. In the current questionnaire, this question was posed at the end. Asking this question at the beginning of the interview will reduce interview time in some cases.

During recruitment no other major issues with the eligibility criteria were noted that would need to be changed in view of a larger follow-up study.

The randomization procedure used in this pilot study did not give each subject an equal chance to get into each intervention group. Computerized block randomization is suggested for the follow-up study (Roberts and Torgerson, 1998).

General administration and organization time before and after the subjects' visit can be reduced. It is recommended to implement a short web-based questionnaire in the recruitment phase prior to the structured telephone interview, in order to pre-screen potential trial participants for eligibility. The use of email and electronic documents for communication is also recommended. This was not considered at the beginning of this pilot study, but was implemented at the request of the subjects.

The use of electronic communication in the pilot study posed an unforeseen problem. Probably due to different printing and scanning settings, the SF-MPQ (t3) form resized. This caused the final printed SF-MPQ (t3) to be different than the original and this had an influence on the length of the VAS, which no longer had the standardized length of 100 mm (Bloomfield and Hanks 1981) (Snow and Kirwan, 1988). The investigator noticed this during the data processing, and chose to adjust in cases where the VAS did not measure the uniform length of 100 mm, by recalculating the data using the rule of 3 – i.e. dividing the length of the indicated distance by the actual length of the VAS scale and multiplying it by 10. To reduce measurement error, it is suggested that a printed copy of the SF-MPQ (t3) be handed to the subject before he or she returns home. Having the subjects return the document by scanning and sending, for the investigator to print out on receipt, might still distort the length of the VAS. However, the baseline will then be the same for everyone and the 3-step calculation will give a more precise comparable result.

Printing and scanning the documents also proved to be an issue for one subject who did not have a functional scanner and printer at home. This was failed to return the SF-MPQ (t3). Clear communication with the subjects prior to the study as regards to handling and the importance of returning questionnaires on time should be foreseen in the follow-up study (Edwards, 2010).

Regarding the subjects' comprehension and completion of the STAI Y-1, Y-2 and SF-MPQ questionnaires, the investigator noted no problems, so this part of the study can be repeated as such. The investigator nevertheless wishes to stipulate that none of the subjects were native English speakers and that this might have influenced their interpretation of the STAI questions. This might also have been the case with the understanding of the descriptions of the qualities of pain in the SF-MPQ (Hawker, et al. 2011).

HRV measurements were taken with the HRV-scanner from the company Biosign®. The position of the electrodes and a single artefact in a 5-minute recording can influence the results (Biosign, 2012) and so this was carefully monitored by the investigator. To ensure a good signal was received the investigator made a visual inspection of the heart rate trace and biosignal on the computer display prior to the 5-minute rest period. When a poor signal was received the investigator optimized the settings of the heart beat detection (Biosign, 2012) or, if needed, changed the position of the electrodes. When electrodes needed to be readjusted, new ones were used. After the five-minute recordings the quality wizard provided by the Biosign® software was used. When insufficient data quality was reported, the artefacts were corrected manually as outlined in the documentation provided with the BioSign® HRV-scanner (Biosign®, 2012) and accepted by the Task Force of The European Society of Cardiology and The North American Society of Pacing and Electrophysiology (1996).

A weakness of HRV measurement is that it is very sensitive. As mentioned above one artefact in a five-minute recording can influence the result. Respiratory parameters, like reductions or increases in respiratory frequency can have an impact on the heart rate oscillations and RR complex (Billman, 2011) (Quintana and Heathers, 2014). In this study respiration was not controlled and might therefore have affected the HRV results. This was probably the case for subject 13, who spontaneously mentioned at the end of the visit having practiced a breathing exercise during the rest period and consequent HRV reading at t1. She didn't practice this at t2.

Other factors that can influence HRV are the use of medication, intake of caffeine, alcohol, food and hydration (Quintana and Heathers, 2014). These factors were addressed in the ICF and verified during the pre-treatment interview.

However, the time of day of the intervention or the explicit instruction to empty the bladder as recommended by Quintana and Heathers (2014) weren't included in this pilot study. These are recommended for inclusion in the follow-up study.

Five-minute HRV recordings, due to their sensitivity, can provide only prognostic information (Task Force of The European Society of Cardiology and The North American Society of Pacing and Electrophysiology,1996).

EDA measurements were carried out with the MentalBioScreen 'K3' device on the non-dominant hand. In this pilot study 14 subjects were right-handed and 1 was left-handed. Before placing the electrodes, the subjects were asked to wash their hands. However this might have influenced the results. Washing with soap is not recommended as it can swell the epidermis (Boucsein, et al. 2012) and should be avoided in the follow-up study.

Corneal hydration is very important and to keep it optimal it is recommended to regulate humidity and temperature in the room (Boucsein, et al. 2012). In this pilot study humidity and temperature were recorded but not regulated. For group B the temperature in the treatment room at t1 between subjects varied from min 21°C to max 23°C and humidity min 45% to max 63%. For group HN the temperature in the treatment room at t1 between subjects varied from min 21°C to max 24°C and humidity min 55% to max 75%. For group HNB the temperature in the treatment room at t1 between subjects varied from min 21°C to max 24°C and humidity min 47% to max 66%.

6.2 Discussion of the Results

6.2.1 Autonomic Nervous System

The 'Reaset Approach' has a favorable effect on the autonomic nervous system measured with HRV, but not with EDA. However there is a difference between groups.

6.2.2 Heart Rate Variability

HRV was evaluated through 3 parameters: the standard deviation of RR intervals (SDNN), the standard deviation of points perpendicular to the axis (SD1) and the standard deviation of points along the axis (SD2)

The results, show that a 25 minute Reaset Approach intervention has a measureable effect on HRV. The results further indicate an effect difference between the three groups. The results of the RA intervention for group HNB showed an increase in all parameters in all subjects (SDNN, SD1 and SD2) compared to groups HN and B.

In group B subject 13 SDNN value decreased from 49,46 ± 8,13 to 28,27 ± 10,99 - a difference of -21,19 ms, SD1 value decreased from 21,29 ± 2,84 to 15,63 ± 7,95 - a difference of -5,66 ms and SD2 value decreased from 66,63 ± 11,48 to 36,79 ± 13,59 - a difference of -29,84 ms. SD2 value also decreased for subject 11 from 68,843 ± 11,48 to 66,85 ± 13,59 - a difference of -1,99 ms.

In group HN subject 15 SDNN value decreased from 33,32 ± 13,38 to 32,08 ± 35,58 - a difference of -1,24 ms and SD2 value decreased from 43,53 ± 12,94 to 38,41 ± 46,86 - a difference of 5,12 ms. Subjects 12 SD1 value decreased from 13,01 ± 16,83 to 11,79 ± 19,6 - a difference of -1,22 ms and subjects 14 SD1 value decreased from 24,84 ± 16,83 to 23,47 ± 19,6 - a difference of -1,37 ms.

Subject 13 from group B, whose SDNN, SD1 and SD2 values decreased, reported at the end of the visit that she had practiced a relaxing meditation exercise in the 10 minutes before the treatment (t1) but not in the period after the treatment where the second measurement was done (t2). This relaxation exercise might have influenced the results (Peng, et al. 2004).

The results are consistent with the findings of Giles et al. (2013), who evaluated an sub-occipital decompression technique on 19 subjects compared to a sham and a time control condition. In their study, SDNN increased significantly in the OMT intervention compared to the sham and time control condition. Henley et al (2008) demonstrated the association between OMT and the ANS in 17 healthy subjects. In their study they compared a cervical myofascial OMT with a touch-only sham OMT and a no-touch control with the subjects in a sympathetic environment (tilt). Only when the OMT was performed was there enough vagal response to overcome the sympathetic tone.

The results are also in line with findings by Moraska et al. (2008), who reviewed physiological adjustments to stress measures following massage. The review included 25 studies and concluded that there was a consistent pre-post reduction in heart rate after a single treatment. These results were in line with a meta-analysis of massage therapy by Moyer, Rounds and Hannum (2004).

6.2.3 ELECTRO-DERMAL ACTIVITY

EDA was reduced in 2 out of 5 subjects (1,11) in group B, in all subjects in group HN and in 4 out of 5 subjects in group HNB (2,4,7,9). All reductions are by less than 1μs. These results are in line with a preliminary investigation by Milnes and Moran (2007), who measured the influence of a CV4 on EDA. The measured data in group B show that EDA increased by more than 1μs in subject 5 and 6.

Most subjects had a very low tone during the whole measurement and it should be questioned whether this test was done properly or influenced by the hand-washing prior to the placing of the electrodes (Boucsein, et al. 2012). Further research is needed in view of a follow-up study.

6.2.4 ANXIETY

There is a preliminary indication that the 'Reaset Approach' has a measurable effect difference pre-post intervention and between the 3 intervention groups in state and trait anxiety.

6.2.4.1 STATE ANXIETY

State anxiety was reduced in all 15 subjects and is in line with the results of another osteopathy study by Dugailly et al. (2014). The results are also comparable with the findings by Lindgren et al. (2013), who evaluated the effect of Touch Massage, and Hatayama et al. (2008), who tested the effect of a facial massage on the ANS and STAI.

There is no evidence, however, that the reduction is due to the intervention itself. Reduction in anxiety can be due to the subject being touched (Jackson, et al. 2008) (Field, 2014), the result of a placebo effect or due to reduction of the distressing symptoms (Williams, 2007). This improvement could also be ascribable to HRV regulation (Friedman, 2007).

6.2.4.2 TRAIT ANXIETY

Trait anxiety improved in all subjects in group B and HN, while in the HNB group one subject demonstrated no change, while another subject's trait anxiety score actually increased. It is very difficult to prove that these results are in fact related to the intervention. The effect on trait anxiety is probably more significant after multiple treatments (Moraska and Chandler, 2009).

6.2.5 MUSCULOSKELETAL PAIN

The 'Reaset Approach' has given preliminary indication for a measurable difference in musculoskeletal pain pre-post intervention and between the 3 intervention groups.

The results of this pilot study are in line with general clinical outcomes associated with osteopathy (Licciardone, Gamber and Cardelli, 2002).

Pain intensity measured with a VAS was reduced in all subjects immediately after the intervention except for subject 6 in group B. Although pain increased again for some subjects in the days following the intervention, 3 days after the intervention pain intensity levels were lower compared to before the intervention.

Total SF-MPQ scores improved in 13 subjects and stayed the same for 1 subject in groups B and HN. Similar to the VAS scores, total SF-MPQ went up slightly again in the days after the treatment but 3 days after the intervention they were still lower than at onset except for 1 subject in group HNB (4) for whom there was no change.

In this pilot study, three different treatment approaches were compared. The preliminary result shows a tendency for of a better outcome in pain intensity in the groups that included the head and neck intervention (HN and HNB). There is insufficient scientific evidence that cranial manipulation has any effect (Green, et al. 1999) or else results have been inconclusive (Jäkel and von Hauenschild, 2011). This being noted, most studies addressing osteopathy in the cranial field have focused on quality of life, sleeping habits, gross motor function, autonomic nervous system functioning and headaches (Jäkel and von Hauenschild, 2011) and not on musculoskeletal pain. Further research into the effect of cranial oriented approaches on musculoskeletal pain is needed

6.3 SUGGESTIONS FOR FUTURE RESEARCH

Musculoskeletal pain is the most common reason for patients to visit an osteopath (Johnson and Kurtz, 2002). In the case of work-related musculoskeletal pain there is growing evidence that psychosocial factors are at the base of these problems rather than biomechanical factors (Mcfarlane, et al., 2009). At the same time as this mind-body link is gaining attention, there is also a growing interest in the body-mind aspects of osteopathy - in other words how osteopathy, as a physical treatment, influences psychosocial aspects of health and wellbeing (Williams, 2007).

This pilot study, which forms the basis of a larger study, gave indication that patients with work-related musculoskeletal pain perceived less pain and less state anxiety after a single treatment.

For a follow-up study it is suggested to monitor the psychosocial and physical benefits over the complete duration of the study. Accordingly, it is recommended to add the numeric rating scale for perceived job stress, which was part of the structured interview and the STAI Y-1 form, 3 days and 21 days after the treatment, and the SF-MPQ again 21 days after the treatment. This will give valuable insights into the lasting psychosocial and physical effect of the Reaset Approach following a single treatment.

Follow-up studies with multiple treatments are recommended to determine the long-term effects of the Reaset Approach on work-related stress levels, musculoskeletal pain and trait anxiety.

7 CONCLUSION

This pilot study determined that a follow-up study with a larger number of subjects can proceed subject to minor modifications.

It is suggested is to conduct the study in several languages, with French as the first alternative to English. This will make it easier to recruit more subjects to have a more representative sample of the actual population of the place where the study is conducted.

In the recruitment phase, the imperative need to meet the three inclusion criteria – namely age between 30 and 50, perceived work-related stress and presence of musculoskeletal pain - should be more strongly stressed.

More attention should be paid to the implications of using electronic documents. Subjects should be explicitly asked if this method of communication is suitable or if regular mail is preferred. To avoid errors with the VAS, it is recommended to give subjects a printed copy of the SF-MPQ before they leave. This will give more accurate comparable results, given the distortion of the scale after scanning and printing.

Further investigation should be conducted into the proper use of the MentalBioScreen 'K3' device.

The preliminary results as regards treatment effect indicate a measureable effect difference pre-post intervention and between groups on the autonomic nervous system (HRV), state and trait anxiety and musculoskeletal pain. The intervention groups that included the head and neck intervention demonstrated better results that the body-only intervention.

The results in treatment effect in this study are promising and an invitation for further research into the body-mind influences of body-based practices. The results also invite further investigation in the biopsychosocial model and the inclusion of body-based practices in non-physical complaints.

8 LITERATURE

AACOM, Glossary of osteopathic terminology, November 2011 edition, URL: http://www.aacom.org/resources/bookstore/Documents/GOHN011ed.pdf, (Accessed: 23. 10.2013).

Alvares, G.A., Quintana, D.S., Kemp, A.H., Van Zwieten, A., Balleine, B.W., et al. (2013). Reduced Heart Rate Variability in Social Anxiety Disorder: Associations with Gender and Symptom Severity. *PLoS ONE* 8 (7), e70468.

Andersen, J.H., Fallentin, N., Thomsen, J.F., Mikkelsen, S. (2011). Risk Factors for Neck and Upper Extremity Disorders among Computers Users and the Effect of Interventions: An Overview of Systematic Reviews. *PLos ONE* 6(5), e19691.

Bach, D.R. (2014). Sympathetic nerve activity can be estimated from skin conductance responses — A comment on Henderson et al. (2012). *Neuroimage* 84 (100), 122–123.

Barnes, L. L. B., Harp, D., Jung, W. S. (2002). Reliability generalization of scores on the Spielberger State–Trait Anxiety Inventory. *Educational and Psychological Measurement, 62,* 603–618.

Billman, G.E. (2011). Heart rate variability – a historical perspective. *Frontiers in Physiology* 2 (86).

Biosign (2012). Documentation for HRV-Scanner V 3.1. Available at http://www.biosign .de/hrv-scanner/downloads/

Black, P.H., Garbutt, L.D. (2001). Stress, inflammation and cardiovascular disease. *Journal of Psychosomatic Research* 52 (1), 1-23.

Bloomfield, S.S., Hanks, G.W. (1981). The visual analogue scale. *British Journal of Clinical Pharmacology* 11 (1).

Boucsein, W., Fowles, D.C., Grimnes, S., Gershon, B., Roth, W.T., Dawson, M.E., Filion, D.L. (2012). Publication recommendations for electrodermal measurements. *Psychophysiology* 49 (8), 1017-1034.

Brosschot, J. F., Van Dijk, E., & Thayer, J. F. (2007). Daily worry is related to low heart rate variability during waking and the subsequent nocturnal sleep period. *International Journal of Psychophysiology* 63 (1), 39-47.

Chalmers, J.A., Quintana, D.S., Abbott, M., M-J., Kemp, A.H. (2014). Anxiety disorders are associated with reduced heart rate variability: a meta-analysis. *Frontiers in Psychiatry* 5 (80).

Chandola, T., Herclides, A., Kumari, M. (2010) Psychophysiological biomarkers of workplace stressors. *Neuroscience Biobehavioral Review* 35 (1), 51-57.

Chandola, T., Britton, A., Brunner, E., Hemingway, H., Malik, M., Kumari, M;, Badrick, E., Kivimaki, M., Marmot, M. ((2008). Work stress and coronary heart disease: What are the mechanisms? *European Heart Journal* 29, 640-648.

Dugailly, P., Fassin, S., Maroye, L., Evers, L., Klein, P., Feiper, V. (2014). Effect of general osteopathic treatment on body satisfaction, global self-perception and anxiety: A randomized trial in asymptomatic female students. *International journal of Osteopathic medicine* 17, 94-101.

Edwards, P. (2010). Questionnaires in clinical trials: guidelines for optimal design and administration. *Trials* 11 (2).

European Agency for Safety and Health at work (EU-OSHA): Brun, A., Milczarek, M., (2007). *Expert forecast on Emerging Psychosocial Risks Related to Occupational Safety and health.* (PDF) Luxembourg office for Official Publications of the European Communities. https://osha.europa.eu/en/publications/reports/7807118 (15 January 2014, date last accessed).

European Agency for Safety and Health at work (EU-OSHA): Milczarek, M., Schneider, E., Gonzalez, E.,R., (2009). *OSH in figures: stress at work - fact and figures.* (PDF) Luxembourg office for Official Publications of the European Communities. https://osha.europa.eu/en/publications/reports/TE-81-08-478-EN-C_SH_ in_ figures_stress_at_work (15 December 2013, date last accessed)

European Foundation for the Improvement of Living and Working Conditions (Eurofound) (2007). Work-related stress. http://www.eurofound.europa.eu/ewco/reports/TN0502TR 01/ TN0502TR01.pdf

Field, T. (2014) Massage therapy research review. *Complimentary therapies in Clinical practices.* (Accepted for publication and published online August 01, 2014)

Fieuw, L., Ott, M. (2005). *Osteopatische techniken im viszeralen bereich.* Stuttgart: Hippokrates.

Finestone, H.M., Alfeeli, A., Fisher, W.A. (2008). Stress-induced Physiologic Changes as a Basis for the Biopsychosocial Model of Chronic Musculoskeletal Pain: A New Theory? *Clinical Journal of Pain* 24 (9).

Friedman, B.H. (2007). An autonomic flexibility-neurovisceral integration model of anxiety and cardiac vagal tone. *Biological Psychology* 74, 185-199.

Gatchel, R.J., Peng, Y.B., Peters, M.L., Fuchs, P.N., Turk, D.C. (2007). The biopsychosocial approach to chronic pain: Scientific advances and future directions. *Psychological Bulletin* 133 (4), 581–624.

Giles, P.D., Hensel, K.L., Pacchia, C.F., Smith, M.L. (2013). Suboccipital Decompression enhances heart rate variability indices of cardiac control in healthy subjects. *The Journal of Alternative and Complimentary Medicine* 19 (2), 92-96.

Griffiths, K.L., Mackey, M.G., Adamson, B.J. (2007). The impact of computerised work environment on professional occupational groups and behavioral and physiological risk factors for musculoskeletal symptoms: A literature review. *Journal of Occupational Rehabilitation* 17, 743-765.

Green, C., Martin, C.W., Bassett, K., Kazanjian, A., (1999). A systematic review of craniosacral therapy: biological plausibility, assessment reliability and clinical effectiveness. *Complimentary Therapies in Medicine* 7 (4), 201-207.

Grisberger, W., Bänzinger, U., Lingg, G., Lothaller, H., Endler,

P.C. (2014). Heart rate variability and the influence of craniosacral therapy on autonomous nervous system regulation in persons with subjective discomforts: a pilot study. *Journal of Integrative Mecidine* 12(3), 156-161.

Groth-Marnat, G. (2003). *Handbook of Psychological Assessment*. 4. Hoboken, NJ: John Wiley.

Hallman, D.M., Olsson, E.M.G., von Schéele, B., Melin, L ., Lyskov, E. (2011). Effects of heart rate variability biofeedback in subjects with stress-related chronic neck pain : A pilot study. *Applied Psychophysiology and Biofeedback* 36, 71-80.

Hallman, D.M., Ekman, A.H., Lyskov, E. (2013). Changes in physical activity and heart rate variability in chronic neck-shoulder pain: monitoring during work and leisure time. *International Archives of Occupational and Environmental health.* Epub ahead of print.

Hansen, A.L., Johnson, B.H., Thayer, J.F. (2003). Vagal influence on working memory and attention. *International Journal of Psychophysiology* 48, 263–274.

Hartvigsen, J., Lings, S., Leboeuf-Yde, C., Bakketeig, L. (2004). Psychosocial factors at work in relation to low back pain and consequences of low back pain; a systematic, critical review of prospective cohort studies. *Occupational and Environmental Medicine* 61 (1).

Hatayama, T., Kitamura S., Tamura, C., Nagano, M., Ohnuku, K. (2008). The facial massage reduced anxiety and negative mood status, and decreased sympathetic nervous activity. *Biomedical Research* 29 (6), 317-320.

Hawker, G.A., Mian, S., Kendzerska, T., Frech, M. (2011) Measurements of adult pain. Visual Analog Scale for Pain (VAS Pain), Numeric Rating Scale for Pain (NRS Pain), McGill Pain Questionnaire (MPQ), Short-Form McGill Pain Questionnaire (SF-MPQ), Chronic Pain Grade Scale (CPGS), Short Form-36 Bodily Pain Scale (SF-36 BPS), and Measure of Intermittent and Constant Osteoarthritis Pain (ICOAP). *Arthritis Care and*

Research 63 (S11), S240-S252.

Henley, C.E., Ivins, D., Mills, M., Wen, F.K., Benjamin, B.A. (2008). Osteopathic manipulative treatment and its relationship to autonomic nervous system activity as demonstrated by heart rate variability: a repeated measures study. *Osteopathic Medicine and primary Care* 2 (7).

Hjortskov, N., Rissen, D., Blangsted, A. K., Fallentin, N., Lundberg, U., & Sogaard, K. (2004). The effect of mental stress on heart rate variability and blood pressure during computer work. *European Journal of Applied Physiology* 92 (1-2), 84-89.

Jackson, E., Kelley, M., McNeil, P., Meyers, P., Schlegel, L., Eaton, M. (2008) Does touch therapy reduce pain and anxiety in patients with cancer? *Clinical Journal of Oncology Nursing* 12 (1), 113-120.

Jäkel, A., von Hauenschild, P. Therapeutic Effects of Cranial Osteopathic Manipulative Medicine: A Systematic Review. *The Journal of the American Osteopathic Association* 111 (12), 685-693.

Jarczok, M.N., Jarczok, M., Mauss, D., Koenig, J., Li, J., Herr, R.M., Thayer J.F. (2013). Autonomic nervous system activity and workplace stressors - A systematic review. *Neuroscience and Behavioral Reviews* 37, 1810-1823.

Jensen, C., Ryholt, C.U., Burr, H., Villadsen, E., Christensen, H. (2002). Work-related psychosocial, physical and individual factors associated with musculoskeletal symptoms in computer users. *Work & Stress* 16, 107-120.

Johnson, S.M., Kurtz, M.E. (2002). Conditions and diagnoses for which osteopathic primary care physicians and specialists use osteopathic manipulative treatment. The *Journal of the American Osteopathic Association* 102 (10).

Johnson, B.H., Hansen, A.L. Murison, R., Eid, J., Thayer, J.F. (2012). Heart rate variability and cortisol responses during attentional and working memory tasks in naval cadets. *International Maritime Health* 63 (4), 181-187.

Kang, M. G., Koh, S. B., Cha, B. S., Park, J. K., Woo, J. M., & Chang, S. J. (2004). Association between job stress on heart rate variability and metabolic syndrome in shipyard male workers. *Yonsei Medical Journal* 45 (5), 838-846.

Korte, S.M., Koolhaas, J.M., Wingfield, J.C., McEwen, B.S. (2005). The Darwinian concept of stress: benefits of allostasis and costs of allostatic load and the trade-offs in health and disease. *Neuroscience and Biobehavioral Reviews* 29, 3-38.

Licciardone, J.C., Brimhall, A.K., King, L.N. (2005). Osteopathic manipulative treatment for low back pain: a systematic review and meta-analysis of randomized controlled trials. *BMC Musculoskeletal Disorders* 6 (43).

Licciardone, J.C., Gamber, R., Cardarelli, K. (2002). Patient satisfaction and clinical outcomes associated with osteopathic manipulative treatment. *Journal American Osteopathic Association* 102 (1).

Licciardone, J.C., Minotti, D.E., Gatchel, R.J., Kearns, C.M., Singh, K.P. (2013). Osteopathic Manual Treatment and Ultrasound Therapy for Chronic Low Back Pain: A Randomized Controlled Trial. *Annals of Family Medicine* 11 (2).

Licht, C. M., de Geus, E. J., van Dyck, R., & Penninx, B. W. (2009). Association between anxiety disorders and heart rate variability in The Netherlands Study of Depression and Anxiety (NESDA). *Psychosomatic Medicine* 71(5), 508-518.

Lin, Y.S., Taylor, G. (1998). Effects of therapeutic touch in reducing pain and anxiety in an elderly population. *Integrative Medicine* 1 (4), 155-162.

Lindgren, L., Lehtipalo, S., Winsö, S., Karlsson, M., Wiklund, U., Brulin, C. (2013) Touch massage: a pilot study of a complex intervention. *Nursing in Critical Care* 18 (6), 269-277.

Mcfarlane, A.C. (2007). Stress-related musculoskeletal pain. *Best Practice & Clinical Rheumatology* 21 (3), 549-565.

Macfarlane, G.J., Pallewatte, N., Paudval, P., Blyth, F.M, Coggon, D., Crombez, G., Linton, S., Leino-Arias, P., Silman, A.J.,

Smeets, R.J., van der Windt, D. (2009). Evaluation of work-related psychosocial factors and regional musculoskeletal pain: results from EULAR Task Force. *Annals of the Rheumatic Diseases* 68 (6), 885-891.

McEwen, B. S. (2001). Plasticity of the hippocampus: Adaptation to chronic stress and allostatic load. *Annals of the New York Academy of Science*, 933, 265–277.

Melzack, R. (1987). The Short-Form McGill Pain Questionnaire. *Pain* 30, 191-197.

Merriam-Webster, Reset, URL: http://www.merriam-webster.com/dictionary/reset (Accessed: 23.10.2013).

Merriam-Webster, Ease, URL: http://www.merriam-webster.com/dictionary/ease?show =0&t =1380872063, (Accessed: 23.10.2013).

Metelka, R. (2014). Heart rate variability - current diagnosis of the cardiac autonomic neuropathy. A review. *Biomedical papers of the Medical Faculty of the University Palacký, Olomouc, Czechoslovakia* 158:XX.

Miles, K., Moran, R.W. (2007). Physiological effects of a CV4 cranial osteopathic technique on autonomic nervous system function: A preliminary investigation. *International Journal of Osteopathic Medicine* 10, 8-17.

Moraska, A., Chandler, C. (2009). Changes in Psychological Parameters in Patients with Tension-type Headache Following Massage Therapy: A Pilot Study. *Journal for Manual Therapy* 17 (2), 96-94.

Moraska, A., Pollini, R.A., Boulanger, K., Brooks, M.Z., Teitlebaum, L. (2008). Physiological adjustments to stress measures following massage therapy: A review of the literature. *Evidence-Based Complimentary and Alternative Medicine* 7 (4), 409-4018.

Moyer, C.A., Rounds, J., Hannum, J.W. (2004). A meta-analysis of massage therapy research. *Psychological Bulletin* 130, 3-18.

Oxford, Approach, URL: http//www.oxforddictionaries.com/ definition/english/approach, (Accessed 17/01/2014).

Peng, C.K., Henry, I.C., Mietus, J.E., Hausdorff, J.M., Khalsa, G., Benson, H., Goldberger, A.L. (2004)/ Heart rate dynamics during three forms of meditation. *International Journal of Radiology* 95, 19-27.

Penney, J.N. (2010). The biopsychosocial model of pain and contemporary osteopathic practice. *International Journal of Osteopathic Medicine* 13, 42–47.

Petrowski, K., Herold, U., Joraschky, P., Mück-Weymann, M., Siepmann, M. (2010). The Effects of Psychosocial Stress on Heart Rate Variability in Panic Disorder. *German Journal of Psychiatry* 2, 66-73.

Psikorski, J., Guzik, P. (2005). Filtering poincaré plots. *Computional Methods in Science and Technology* 11 (1), 39-48.

Punnett, L., Bergqvist. U., (1997). Visual display unit work and upper extremity musculoskeletal disorders. A review of epidemiological findings. (National Institute for Working Life - Ergonomic Expert Committee Document No 1). *Arbete och Hälsa* 1-161.

Quintana, D.S., Heathers, J.A.J. (2014). Considerations in the assessment of heart rate variability in biobehavioral research. *Frontiers in Physiology* 5 (805).

Roberts, C., Torgerson, D. (1998). Randomisation methods in controlled trials. *British Medical Journal* 7, 317(7168): 1301-1310.

Scherding, C. (2013). Osteopathie bei Depressionen: Kurzzeiteffekt auf Herzraten-variabilität, befinden und Schweregrad. MSc. Osteopathie Schule Deutschland.

Setz, C., Arnrich, B.A., Schumm, J., La Marca, R. (2010) Discriminating stress from cognitive load using a wearable EDA device. *IEEE Transactions on information technology in Biomedicine* 14 (2), 410-417.

Snow, S., Kirwan, J.R. (1988). Visual analogue scale: a source of error. *Annals of the Rheumatic Disease* 47 (6), 526.

Spielberger, C. D. (1983). *Manual for the State-Trait Anxiety Inventory (Form Y)*. Palo Alto, CA: Mind Garden.

Spielberger, C. D. (1989). State-Trait Anxiety Inventory: A comprehensive bibliography. Palo Alto, CA: Consulting Psychologists Press.

Stolberg, H., Norman, G., Trop, I. (2004). Randomized controlled trials. *American Journal of Roentgenology* 183 (6), 1539-1544.

Strand, L.I., Ljunggren, A.E., Bogen, B., Ask, T., Johnsen, T.B. (2008) The Short-Form McGill Pain Questionnaire as an outcome measure: Test-retest reliability and responsiveness to change. *European Journal of Pain* 12, 917-925.

Task Force of The European Society of Cardiology and The North American Society of Pacing and Electrophysiology (1996). Guidelines: heart rate variability—standards of measurement, physiological interpretation, and clinical use. *Circulation* 93, 1043–1065.

Thayer, J.F., Lane, R.D. (2009). Claude Bernard and the heart–brain connection: Further elaboration of a model of neurovisceral integration. *Neuroscience and Biobehavioral Reviews* 33, 81–88.

Tonello, L., Rodrigues, F., Souza, J.W.S., Campell, C.S.G., Leicht, A.S., Boullosa, D.A. (2014). The role of physical activity and heart rate variability for the control of work related stress. *Frontiers in physiology* 5 (67).

Waersted, M., Hanvold, T.N., Veiersted, K.O. (2010). Computer work and musculoskeletal disorders of the neck and upper extremity: A systematic review. *BMC Musculoskeletal Disorders* 11(79).

Williams, N., (2007). Optimising the psychological benefits of osteopathy. *International Journal of Osteopathic Medicine* 10, 36-41.

Wiktionary, Ease, URL: http://en.wiktionary.org/wiki/ease (access: 23.10.2013).

9 ADDENDUM

9.1 INDEX OF ABBREVIATIONS

ANS	Autonomic nervous system
B	"Body" intervention
BPM	Beats per minute
ECG	Electrocardiogram
EU	European Union
EDA	Electro-dermal activity
HF	Power in high frequency range of HRV (0,15 – 0,4 Hz)
HN	"Head & neck" intervention
HNB	"Head, neck & body" intervention
HRV	Heart rate variability
ICF	Informed consent form
LF	Power in low frequency range of HRV (0,4 – 0,15 Hz)
MS	Millisecond
MS2	Millisecond squared
MSP	Musculoskeletal pain
NN	Normal to normal
NRS	Numeric rating scale
PCF	Patient consent form
PPI	Present pain intensity
PRI	Pain rating index
PSNS	Parasympathetic nervous system
QRS	Combination of 3 of the graphical deflections seen on an ECG
RA	Reaset approach
RR	Interval between R waves from one QRS complex to another
SD	Standard deviation
SD1	Dispersion of points perpendicular to the axis of line-of-identity
SD2	Dispersion of points along the axis of line-of-identity
SDNN	Standard deviation of the RR intervals and index of overall HRV
SEQ	Self-evaluation questionnaire
SF-MPQ	Short-Form McGill Pain Questionnaire
SNS	Sympathetic nervous system
STAI	State-Trait Anxiety Inventory
STAI Y-1	State Anxiety Inventory
STAI Y-2	Trait Anxiety Inventory
t0	Prior to the appointment
t1	Just before the intervention
t2	Immediately after the intervention
t3	3 days after the intervention
t4	21 days after the intervention
VAS	Visual analogue scale
WRS	Work-related stress

9.2 FLOW CHART

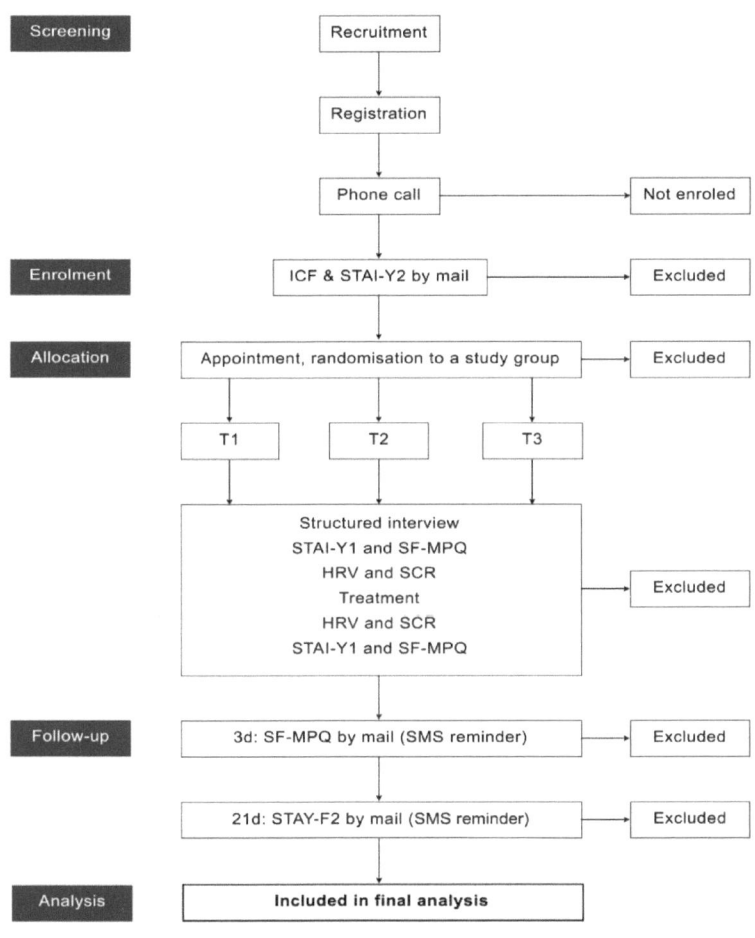

Screening — Recruitment → Registration → Phone call → Not enroled

Enrolment — ICF & STAI-Y2 by mail → Excluded

Allocation — Appointment, randomisation to a study group → Excluded

T1   T2   T3

Structured interview
STAI-Y1 and SF-MPQ
HRV and SCR
Treatment
HRV and SCR
STAI-Y1 and SF-MPQ → Excluded

Follow-up — 3d: SF-MPQ by mail (SMS reminder) → Excluded

21d: STAY-F2 by mail (SMS reminder) → Excluded

Analysis — **Included in final analysis**

9.3 FOLLOW-UP STUDY

To obtain the title: Master of Science in Osteopathy

Date: 2016-2017

Title: The effect of the Reaset Approach on the autonomic nervous system, musculoskeletal pain, state and trait anxiety and perceived stress in office workers: a randomized controlled trial.

Background: Neck-shoulder pain, stress and anxiety have become the most common work-related health problems in office workers in the EU. These symptoms are linked to the increase in psychosocial risks that have emerged with the evolution towards a more computerized work environment.

Objective: To evaluate the effectiveness of a 25 minute 'Reaset Approach' intervention on autonomic regulation evaluated through heart rate variability (HRV), neck-shoulder pain, state and trait anxiety, and perceived stress compared to a control condition.

Methods: 40 office workers with perceived work-related stress and neck-shoulder pain randomly assigned to a control group (rest) or treatment group (Reaset Approach). Trait anxiety and perceived stress questionnaires will be completed pre- and 21-day post-intervention. Resting HRV will be derived in the time-domain pre and post intervention. State anxiety and perceived pain intensity questionnaires will be completed pre-post intervention. Perceived pain intensity will be followed-up 3 and 21-day post intervention.

9.4   ABOUT THE AUTHOR

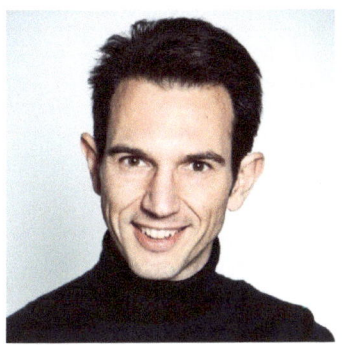

Tom Meyers (1970, Belgium) is an Osteopath D.O., stress coach, public speaker, writer and visionary in the field of health and wellbeing. He runs a private practice in Brussels, Belgium and travels regularly to give presentations and workshops on the topic of 'Understanding & Managing Stress'.

His personal experience and professional insights have led to the development of the 'Reaset Approach', a novel body-mind healing approach and educational system.

Tom is currently conducting the follow-up MSc study and writes his first self-help book.

In his book 'Reaset: The Return of Ease', Tom takes you on a journey where he interlaces soul-purpose, personal development, health and healing into a compelling self-help guide to thrive in times of change and adversity.

Please check out his website for more information on the Reaset Approach, EOD, articles, the follow-up study and upcoming book.

www.reaset.me

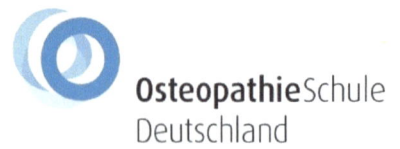

OsteopathieSchule
Deutschland

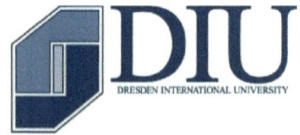

www.ingramcontent.com/pod-product-compliance
Lightning Source LLC
Chambersburg PA
CBHW040826180526
45159CB00001B/81